D1570820

Defects of Secretion in Cystic Fibrosis

ADVANCES IN EXPERIMENTAL MEDICINE AND BIOLOGY

Defects of Secretion in Cystic Fibrosis

Edited by

Carsten Schultz

European Molecular Biology Laboratory
Heidelberg, Germany

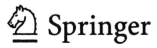 Springer

Library of Congress Cataloging-in-Publication Data

Defects of secretion in cystic fibrosis/edited by Carsten Schultz.
  p.   ; cm. — (Advances in experimental medicine and biology; v. 558)
  Includes bibliographical references and index.
  ISBN 0-387-23076-9 (alk. paper)
    1. Cystic fibrosis—Pathophysiology. 2. Cystic fibrosis—Molecular aspects. I. Schultz,
  Carsten. II. Series.
    [DNLM: 1. Cystic Fibrosis—physiopathology—Congresses. 2. Cystic
  Fibrosis—therapy—Congresses. 3. Cystic Fibrosis Transmembrane Conductance
  Regulator—Congresses. 4. Pancreas—secretion—Congresses. WI 820 D313 2005]
  RC858.C95D44 2005
  616.3'72—dc22

                                                                        2004063217

ISBN: 0-387-23076-9
eISBN: 0-387-23250-8

Printed in the United States of America.   (BS/DH)

9 8 7 6 5 4 3 2 1

springeronline.com

Acknowledgments

I would like to thank Sylke Helbing and Bettina Schäfer for editorial help and Nicole Heath for critically reading through part of the manuscripts. I also would like to acknowledge all speakers and participants of the 'Defects of Secretion' symposium held in Heidelberg in November 2003. Your contributions and lively discussions made the compilation of this book worth while.

Contributing Authors

Gabriele Adam
Universität Regensburg, Germany

Susan J. Anderson
University of Alabama at Birmingham, AL, USA

Tanja Bachhuber
Universität Regensburg, Germany

Dale J. Benos
University of Alabama at Birmingham, AL, USA

Christoph Böhmer
Eberhard-Karls-Universität Tübingen, Germany

Horst Fischer
Children's Hospital Oakland Research Institute, Oakland, CA, USA

Catherine M. Fuller
University of Alabama at Birmingham, AL, USA

Sherif Gabriel
University of North Carolina, Chapel Hill, NC, USA

Erich Gulbins
Eberhard-Karls-Universität Tübingen, Germany

Gunnar C. Hansson
Göteborg University, Gothenburg, Sweden

Jean-Daniel Horisberger
University Lausanne, Switzerland.

Beate Illek
Children's Hospital Oakland Research Institute, Oakland, CA, USA

Malin E. V. Johansson
Göteborg University, Gothenburg, Sweden

Reinhard Kandolf
Eberhard-Karls-Universität Tübingen, Germany

Rolf K.-H. Kinne
Max-Planck-Institut für molekulare Physiologie, Dortmund, Germany

Helmut Kipp
Max-Planck-Institut für molekulare Physiologie, Dortmund, Germany

Karin Klingel
Eberhard-Karls-Universität Tübingen, Germany

Gergely Kovacs
University of Alabama at Birmingham, AL, USA

Karl Kunzelmann
Universität Regensburg, Germany

Florian Lang
Eberhard-Karls-Universität Tübingen, Germany

Albrecht Lepple-Wienhues
Eberhard-Karls-Universität Tübingen, Germany

Martin E. Lidell
Göteborg University, Gothenburg, Sweden

Marcus Mall
The University of North Carolina, Chapel Hill, NC, USA

Mark Moody
Inologic Inc., Seattle, WA, USA

Bettina Mürle
Universität Regensburg, Germany

Paul M. Quinton
UCSD School of Medicine, La Jolla, CA, USA

Monica Palmada
Eberhard-Karls-Universität Tübingen, Germany

Carla M. Pedrosa Ribeiro
The University of North Carolina, Chapel Hill, NC, USA

Andres Ponce
UCSD School of Medicine, La Jolla, CA, USA

Marsh M. Reddy
UCSD School of Medicine, La Jolla, CA, USA

Philippe Roussel
Université de Lille 2, Lille, France

Rainer Schreiber
Universität Regensburg, Germany

Carsten Schultz
European Molecular Biology Laboratory, Heidelberg, Germany

Steve B. Shears
N.I.E.H.S./N.I.H./D.H.S.S., Research Triangle Park, NC, USA

Ildicko Szabo
Eberhard-Karls-Universität Tübingen, Germany

Alexis Traynor-Kaplan
Inologic Inc., Seattle, WA, USA

Frank Thévenot,
Universität Witten/Herdecke, Witten, Germany.

Thilo Voelcker
Universität Regensburg, Germany.

Sabine Wallisch
Eberhard-Karls-Universität Tübingen, Germany

Ling Yang
N.I.E.H.S./N.I.H./D.H.S.S., Research Triangle Park, NC, USA.

Preface

Cystic fibrosis (CF) is the most abundant homocygote inherited disease in the western world. There are about 60,000 patients worldwide. Despite a stable number of new incidents the total number is increasing due the fact that the average lifespan of CF patients has increased from about 8 years in the 1960's to currently over 30 years. Genetic analysis has certainly added patients with mild manifestations who were previously not recognized as CF patients. Overall, however, the increase in life expectancy is mainly due to improved treatment in hospitals and increased knowledge and expertise of physicians around the world. This process has been largely fostered by implementation of CF centers in the US and Europe, where the concentration of required expertise can be more efficiently provided by a team of physicians than in a doctor's practice. The focus, however, needs to expand from the predominantly pediatric level to the treatment of adult patients, a tremendous task for clinics and caretakers. In comparison, the achievements of basic research appear to be very moderate. Laboratories have yet to produce a drug that reverses the basic defect, although several drug candidates that promise increases in chloride secretion and a reduction of the pathologically high sodium uptake of airway epithelia are in clinical trials.

In a meeting, held at the European Molecular Biology Laboratory (EMBL) late in 2003, an international group of scientists gathered to discuss current developments in basic research and novel ways to treat CF. The present volume contains contributions from many of the meeting's speakers and the subjects are wide-ranging encompassing mucus secretion, intracellular epithelial signaling, and the nature and regulation of epithelial ion channels, as well as some of the most recent ideas to prepare CF drug candidates based on intracellular signaling molecules.

Contents

Chapter 1

OUTSIDE NEURONS/INSIDE EPITHELIA: NOVEL ACTIVATION OF CFTR CL⁻ AND HCO₃⁻ CONDUCTANCES

Marsh M. Reddy[1], Andres Ponce[1], and Paul M. Quinton[1,2]
[1]*Department of Pediatrics, UCSD School of Medicine, La Jolla, California 92093-0831;* [2]*Division of Biomedical Sciences, University of California Riverside, Riverside, CA 92021, USA. Phone 001-619-543-2884, fax 001-619-543-568, e-mail: pquinton@ucsd.edu*

1. INTRODUCTION

Cystic Fibrosis (CF) is a disease of abnormal electrolyte transport caused by defects in an anion selective channel, "CFTR". The disease is characterized by poor salt absorption in exocrine ducts, poor cAMP dependent bicarbonate and fluid secretion by pancreas, intestine, and other exocrine epithelia. CF causes an early onset of refractory airway infections that usually eventually result in respiratory failure. The link between the electrolyte transport defect and chronic lung infection remains poorly understood.

The CFTR channel is located specifically in the apical membrane of certain secretory cells and in both luminal and basilateral membranes of absorptive cells.[1] The channel protein is a large complicated structure composed of 1480 amino acids forming 12 transmembrane domains, 2 cytosolic nucleotide binding domains and a cytosolic putatively referred to as regulatory domain because of the numerous consensus phosphorylation sites present in it. The mature protein when expressed in the plasma membrane also exhibits two glycosylated sites on the extracellular surface.

Since the early work of Sato,[2] cAMP activation of protein kinase A mediated phosphorylation has been an accepted and apparently become a universal method for stimulating the CFTR dependent Cl⁻ conductance. In subsequent years, considerable evidence has been presented to demonstrate that activation of the channel usually requires ATP as well as phosphorylation. However, several other mechanisms have also been implicated, which may involve activation by cGMP and/or trimeric G-proteins. When activated in this classic manner, the channel is not only highly conductive to Cl⁻, but also conductive to HCO_3^-, although less so $(PCl^- / PHCO_3^- \sim 0.15)$.

In the course of investigating the permeability of a panel of different anions for CFTR permeability, we were surprised to find that glutamate, renowned for its role in neural synaptic transmission and apparently independent of cAMP and ATP, was a potent activator of CFTR when applied to the cytosolic side of the membrane at low mM concentrations. Moreover, the precursors, α-keto glutarate and glutamine also activated the channel at similar levels of concentration. Equally, surprising we found that even though activation of CFTR by any of these substances caused a rapid and marked increase in Cl⁻ conductance, the channel remained relatively impermeable to HCO_3^-. However, addition of ATP with any of these agonists caused the channel to shift its selectivity and become HCO_3^- conductive.

2.   MATERIALS AND METHODS

2.1   Subjects

Sweat glands were obtained from male volunteers and male patients with Cystic Fibrosis ranging in age from 18 to 57 years. All volunteers gave informed consent to the protocol as approved by the UCSD Internal Review Board for human subjects.

2.2   Biopsy

Generally, four small, full thickness biopsies approximately 1/8" in diameter were removed from the upper back over the scapula and either used immediately or stored at 4°C in NaCl Ringer's solution.

2.3   Dissection

Eccrine sweat glands were identified visually under a dissecting microscope. The coiled portion of the gland, without the straight duct segment, was removed from the collagen matrix of the dermis with fine tipped forceps. Then, under higher magnification (*ca.* 50 X) with trans illumination, a segment of reabsorptive duct of about 1 mm length was carefully dissected from the secretory tubule of the gland using fine insect pins, sharpened forceps, and/or sapphire knives.

2.4 Solutions

Four compositions of Ringer's solutions were used including NaCl, KCl, NaGluconate (NaGlu), KGluconate (KGlu) (all 150 mM) in a basic salt solution containing in addition K^+ (5), Ca^{++} (2), Mg^{++} (1.2), HPO_4^{3-} (3.5), SO_4^{-2} (1.2) titrated to pH 7.4. When applied to the cytosolic compartment, the KGluconate solution was adjusted with NaEDTA (2 mM) to a final Ca^{++} of 8×10^{-8} M and titrated to a final pH of 6.8.

2.5 Microperfusion

Isolated duct segments were then canulated with concentric glass pipettes pulled to tip diameters of approximately 8 microns (inner perfusion pipette) and 30-40 microns (i.d., outer holding pipette) as described earlier (ref). The inner pipette was pulled from septated theta glass (Clark Biomedical Supplies) to form two parallel barrels. One barrel was filled with NaCl (150) and used to inject constant current pulses of 50 nA/ 0.5 sec at 20-second intervals. The other barrel served to perfuse the lumen of the duct with perfusates of choice and to simultaneously record the luminal potential relative to bath (ground).

2.6 BLM Permeabilization

After cannulating and initiating microperfusion with NaGlu in the lumen and validating tissue integrity (only ducts with transepithelial Cl⁻ diffusion potentials more negative than −50 mV were accepted), we changed the bathing solution to 150 KGlu (low Ca^{++} + 5 mM ATP) and exposed the contra luminal surface of the duct to *ca.* 2,000 units/ ml. of α-toxin purified from *Staphylococcus aureus* (CalBiochem). Permeabilization of the BLM occurred over a period of 15-20 minutes and was followed as a progressive increase in transepithelial resistance and decreases in Cl⁻ diffusion potentials to free solution values. After completion of permeabilization, luminal and bathing solutions were changed as needed in the protocol.

2.7   Apical Membrane Anion Selectivity

The apical membrane of the sweat duct exhibits virtually no K^+ conductance and its Na^+ conductance is effective blocked with amiloride.[3] By perifusing and perfusing with K^+ salts or in the presence of the amiloride, the permeabilized duct effectively becomes a single membrane preparation whose conductance is predominantly, if not exclusively (excepting leak pathways) due to anions permeating CFTR. Thus, manipulations that activate the channel are easily visualized as concomitant increases in the magnitude of the anion diffusion potential and transmembrane conductance (Gt). Conductance was calculated from the size of the voltage deflection in response to the current pulse and the microscopically measured diameter of the duct lumen applying the cable equation.[4]

2.8   RT-PCR

We tested for the expression of mRNA for each of eight metabotrophic glutamine receptors (MGR) using primers characteristic of each as follows: **MGR1f** (AGA TGA ACA AGA GTG GAG), **MGR1r** (AAC AAG GTA ACA AGG ATT CCC AGG), **MGR2f** (TGG TGT TAT TGG CGG TTC CTA CAG), **MGR2r** (TCC AGT TGA AGA AGC GGA GAA TC), **MGR3f** (ACT TCA CGG CTC CAT TCA ACC), **MGR3r** (TCA TTT CAT TGG GGG CAC AG), **MGR4f** (ATC GCC CAG TCG GTG AAG ATA C), **MGR4r** (CAG TGG AAG TTG TCC TCC CAG AAC), **MGR5f** (ACA ACC ACA AGA AAC CGA CGA C), **MGR5r** (TGG GAC ACA TTC ACA ACG CCT C), **MGR6f** (ATC CAG ACA ACC ACG CTA ACC G), **MGR6r** (GTT CTT CCA CAC TGC CCA ATC C), **MGR7f** (TGC CGA ATA CTG GGA GGA AAA C), **MGR7r** (CAG GAA GAC AGG AAT CAC AGC C), **MGR8f** (GGA TTG GCT CAG ATA GTT GGG G), **MGR8r** (CAG AGG GCA AAG TTC ACA GGA C).

3.   RESULTS

3.1   Chloride

3.1.1   Classic cAMP/ATP Activation

It is a striking feature of the reabsorptive sweat duct that the CFTR channel under conditions of microperfusion always appears to be constitutively open. That is, initially, upon cannulation and perfusion with a

Cl gradient, almost Nernstian Cl diffusion potentials are presented in the complete absence of exogenous chemical activation.[3,5,6] In fact, in order to inactivate CFTR gCl, the BLM must be permeabilized, during which time CFTR gCl falls to virtually zero, i.e., free solution junction potential (Figure 1). We attributed this deactivation to a loss of cytoplasmic components, putatively cAMP and/ or ATP, necessary to maintain CFTR in the activated state. After permeabilization of the BLM and deactivation of CFTR, gCl was reactivated by adding back cAMP (0.1 mM) plus ATP (5 mM) (Figure 1).

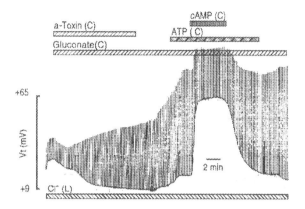

Figure 1. Trace of transepithelial voltage (V_t) of a basilaterally permeabilized, microperfused human sweat duct. The bottom of the curve indicates the voltage (mV) due to the lumen to bath Cl gradient. Upward deflections indicate repetitive constant current pulses. Increases in V_t and smaller pulse deflections indicate greater CFTR Cl conductance. Classically, after permeabilization (left), both cAMP and ATP must be added to the cytosol to activate CFTR (acute rise in V_t, right). Upon withdrawing cAMP, the Cl conductance begins to shut down even in the presence of ATP (slow decline in V_t). In the absence of ATP, cAMP cannot activate CFTR (not shown).

3.1.2   Activation by Glutamate Precursor Amino Acids

After permeabilization and deactivation of CFTR gCl, addition of as little as 1 mM glutamate, will reactivate CFTR gCl (Figures 2,3). Figure 4 shows the response of CFTR gCl to two precursors of glutamate, α-keto glutarate and glutamine. In excellent preparations, either α-keto glutarate or glutamate concentrations as low as 1 mM produced almost the same average gCl response as when activated with cAMP+ATP. None of these compounds were effective when applied to the extracellular surface in the lumen. In contrast, even at isotonic concentrations when we added aspartate or taurine (Figure 5) or D-glutamate, glucuronate, cyclamate, GABA, and, of course, gluconate to the cytoplasm, there was no increase in CFTR gCl. Glucose (10 mM) was without effect.

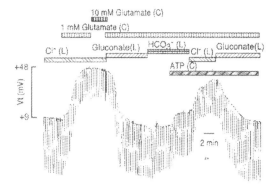

Figure 2. Trace of transepithelial voltage (V_t) of a basilaterally permeabilized, microperfused human sweat duct. The top of the curve indicates the voltage (mV) due to the lumen to bath Cl- gradient and to continual constant current pulses. Increases in V_t and smaller current pulse deflections indicate greater CFTR Cl⁻ conductance. Classically, after permeabilization (left), both cAMP and ATP must be added to the cytosol to activate CFTR (acute rise in V_t). Upon withdrawing cAMP, the Cl⁻ conductance begins to shut down even in the presence of ATP (slow decline in V_t). However, after removing both cAMP and ATP, addition of glutamate to the cytoplasm causes renewed activation of CFTR-gCl (2nd rise in V_t), which reverses when glutamate is withdrawn (2nd fall in V_t). Note that the maximum CFTR response to glutamate is equal to that of classic cAMP/ATP activation.

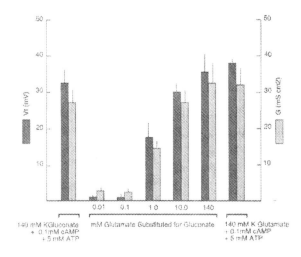

Figure 3. Glutamate at concentrations of 0.1 mM or below did not activate CFTR. Maximal activation appeared to be achieved by about 10 mM and adding cAMP plus ATP did not cause any additional increase in total conductance (G_t).

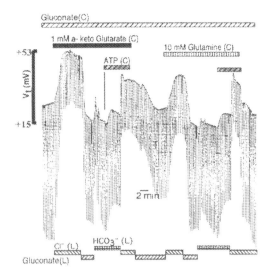

Figure 4. Adding low mM concentrations of either α-keto glutarate or glutamine, precursors for glutamate, also activates CFTR-gCl. Note that there is no HCO_3^- conductance until ATP is added.

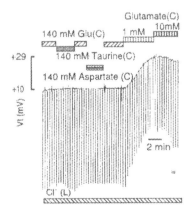

Figure 5. Examples of the lack of effect of taurine and aspartate in contrast to the effect of 1mM glutamate on activating CFTR gCl are shown. Other small anions and amino acids were similarly without effect (cf. text).

3.1.3   No ATP Required

Adding back ATP (5 mM) without cAMP is inadequate for activating CFTR (Figure 1),[7] but activation of CFTR-gCl by any of these three precursors did not require ATP. Furthermore, adding ATP (5mM) or ATP plus cAMP (0.1 mM) did not increase gCl⁻ over gCl⁻ maximally activated with glutamate (Figure 3). This fact alone argues that glutamate and its precursors are not acting as substrates for ATP production.

3.1.4   No Phosphorylation Required

To test whether any mechanism of phosphorylation might be required in this activation, we treated the tissue with general non-specific kinase inhibitor, Staurosporine (10^{-6} M).[8] As seen in Figure 6, staurosporine did not block the response to glutamate.

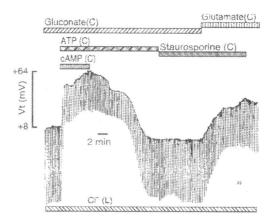

Figure 6. General inhibition of kinases with the promiscuous inhibitor, staurosporine, had no detectable effect on the activation of CFTR gCl with glutamate.

3.2 HCO_3^-

3.2.1   Dynamic HCO_3^- Selectivity

Even though CFTR conducts both Cl^- and HCO_3^- when activated classically with cAMP/ATP, it only conducts Cl^- and remains impermeable to HCO_3^- when activated by glutamate or its precursors (Figure 7 and Figure 4).

3.2.2   ATP Required

However, upon adding 5 mM ATP in the presences of these agonists, CFTR became conductive to HCO_3^- as well (Figure 7). Hydrolyzable ATP was necessary to change the CFTR anion selectivity from impermeable to permeable to HCO_3^-. The non-hydrolysable ATP analogue AMP-PNP ($\bar{\beta}\gamma$-

imidoadenosine 5'-phosphate) did not support HCO_3^- conductance (Figure 8). The activation was dose dependent on cytosolic ATP. At 1.0 mM, ATP produced only about 50% of that induced by physiological concentrations of intracellular ATP (5 mM). Slight increases were sometimes observed at 0.1 mM, but no conductance was detected at 0.01 mM (Figure 9).

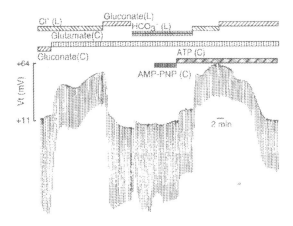

Figure 7. After activating CFTR with glutamate, addition of the poorly hydrolyzable ATP analog, AMP-PNP, did not induce HCO_3^- conductivity. However, it promptly appeared upon replacing the analog with ATP. (C = cytoplasmic; L = luminal).

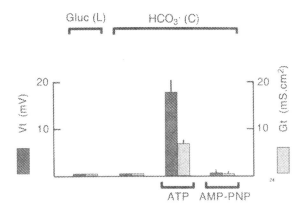

Figure 8. When activated with glutamate, ATP (5.0 mM) increased both the HCO_3^- diffusion potential ($VHCO_3^-$) and conductance ($gHCO_3^-$) whereas the poorly hydrolyzable analog AMP-PNP at the same concentration had no effect on either. (Gluc = gluconate; C = cytoplasmic; L = luminal).

3.2.3   No Phosphorylation Required

Like glutamate-activated gCl, however, phosphorylation did not appear to be required for the activation of the HCO_3^- conductance. Again, staurosporine had no effect on the increase in ATP dependent HCO_3^- conductance.

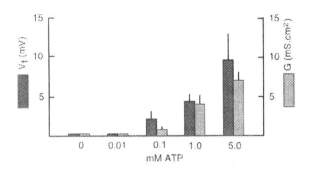

Figure 9. Dose response of CFTR $gHCO_3^-$ to increasing concentrations of ATP. Responses to 1.0 and 5 mM were statistically different from zero ($p < 0.05$).

3.3   Glutamate Receptors

Since glutamate acts through well-described receptors in the neural system, we tested for the possible presence of metabotrophic glutamate receptors in the sweat duct by RT-PCR. In a survey with primers unique for each of eight known receptors, we identified two possible receptor candidates for glutamate in the sweat duct. Metabotrophic receptors (MGR) 3 and 4 appear to be expressed in the sweat gland. MGR3 gave a predicted band at 240 bp, which appeared clearly along with predicted product bands for CFTR, ENaC, and β-actin used controls. MGR4 was only detectable by direct visualization of the fluorescing gel (Figure 10).

3.4   Evidence of CFTR Activation

It is of no small concern that the observed glutamate activation of gCl and ATP dependent activation of $gHCO_3^-$ may be due to activation of an anion channel or channels distinct from CFTR. We tested this possibility by selecting sweat ducts from patients with cystic fibrosis with known genotypes. Ducts were obtained from 3 patients homozygous for the most common CF defect, ΔF508, in which mutant CFTR is not processed to the plasma membrane.[9] In these ducts, glutamate did not increase the Cl⁻ diffusion potential or gCl, nor did glutamate + ATP increase either parameter (Figure 11).

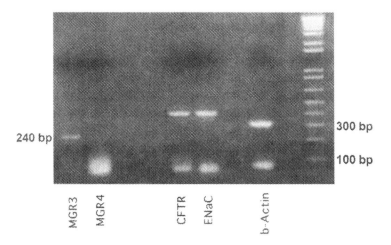

Figure 10. Ethedium bromide stained gel of RT-PCR products for MGR3 (lane 1), MGR4 (240 bp, lane 2), CFTR (420 bp, lane 3), ENaC (410 bp, lane 4), β-actin (300 bp, lane 5), and 100 bp ladder (lane 6). MGR4 appeared as a faint band, not detectable in the transposed figure.

On the other hand, when we examined ducts from two patients with heterozygous genotypes (R117H/ΔF508), gCl was about 15% of normal ducts when stimulated with glutamate, but gHCO3 was about 50% of normal ducts when stimulated with glutamate + ATP (Figure 11).

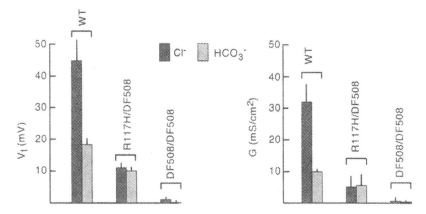

Figure 11. Microperfused ducts from three genotypes of CFTR all show significantly different diffusion potential (V_t; left panel) and conductance (G_t; right panel) responses for Cl- (blue) and HCO_3^- (green) when activated by glutamate or glutamate plus ATP, respectively. (Homozygous normal = WT; heterozygous CF= R117H /ΔF508; homozygous CF = ΔF508/ΔF508.)

4.   4. DISCUSSION

4.1   Excitation by Glutamate and Precursors

4.1.1   Required Concentrations

We have previously reported that Glutamate stimulated CFTR activity with an estimated EC50 of about 3 mM.[10] However, we find now that in some preparations, the concentration needed for this activation may be even lower. Figure 2 shows an example of a preparation in which apparently maximal glutamate activation was achieved at approximately 1 mM. In general, responses did not increase significantly when the cytoplasmic levels were increased from 10 to 140 mM glutamate (Figure 3). Furthermore, α-keto glutarate, which forms glutamate by amination via glutamate dehydrogenase (EC 1.2.4.2; Figure 12), was also capable of activating CFTR gCl at equally low concentrations (Figure 4). Likewise, glutamine, which forms glutamate by deamination by glutaminase (EC 3.5.1.2; Figure 12), can also activate the channel at low mM concentrations (Figure 4). All of these compounds may exist at mM concentrations in the cell. Intracellular glutamate has been reported at about 10 mM in rat tissues[11] and more than 20 mM in human endothelial cells.[12] Our findings here may suggest an alternative explanation for the constitutive activity of CFTR in the sweat duct. That is, it may be cytosolic levels of glutamate (or a precursor) that keeps the channel open. Upon permeabilizing the BLM, small solutes of molecular weight of up to 5,000 are lost from the cell.[13] It may be this loss and not necessarily, as we previously surmised, the loss of cAMP and/or ATP, that deactivates the channel when the cell membrane is permeabilized. This implies that in the duct, the physiologic regulation of CFTR may be under the control of cytoplasmic components other than protein kinase A and ATP.

4.1.2   Modes of Action

Since these compounds are inter convertible and can enter the citric acid cycle via α–keto glutarate (Figure 12), a first thought might be that these substances are simply acting as a source for energy production. However, several pieces of evidence argue against such a conclusion. First, we used other substrates that could have also been used for energy sources with no effect. Second, since classic activation of CFTR requires cytoplasmic concentrations of ATP ($\approx$ 5mM) for maximal activation,[7,14] we question whether such concentrations of ATP could be accumulated in the permeabilized duct cells, especially from substrate concentrations as low as

1 mM. Third, the fact that exogenously added ATP even at 5 mM concentration does not activate CFTR without cAMP, while glutamate at 1mM alone can activate CFTR, speaks strongly against the possibility that ATP is being synthesized de novo from these substances.

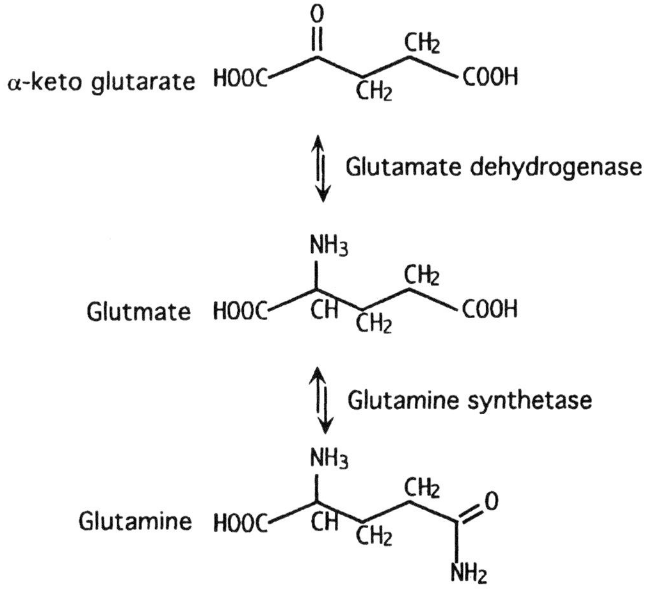

Figure 12. Structures and inter conversion reaction of glutamate and its precursors, α-keto glutarate and glutamine. All are five carbon chain carboxylic acids, but are diverse in amino and carboxyl groups as well as net charge (from –2 to +1).

4.1.3   Kinase Activation

A second thought is that glutamate might be converted to ATP (or precursors) and simultaneously activate an intracellular kinase that activates CFTR by phosphorylation. (Kinases such as PKA require nM-μM concentrations of ATP, which might be formed from these substrates.[15,16]) Thus, if CFTR requires phosphorylation to activate with glutamate, it must take place via a kinase that is insensitive to the promiscuous kinase inhibitor, staurosporine. We have shown previously that staurosporine blocks cAMP/ATP activation of CFTR,[17,18] but as seen in Figure 6, staurosporine did not inhibit the effect of glutamate. Thus, the possibilities that glutamate may act via another intracellular pathway (it has no effect extracellularly) or may act directly on CFTR must be entertained. Suggestive of an intracellular pathway, we found evidence of two metabotrophic glutamate receptors #3 and #4 by RT-PCR, although only MGR3 product appeared definitively as a strong band (Figure 10). At present, we do not know if this receptor has any role in the present phenomenon.

4.1.4   Ligand Binding

If these metabolites are not acting by virtue of ATP production, they may be acting as a ligand(s) for an intracellular receptor or directly on CFTR per se. Although the structures of these agonists are related as 5-carbon carboxy acid chains, they are diverse in net charge and amino groups. The amine of C-2 can be replaced by an ester, and the -OH of C-5 can be replaced by an amine. This disparity may argue that only one form actually participates in stimulating CFTR and that the others are precursors that are enzymatically converted into it.   To determine whether direct interaction with and activation of CFTR occurs likely will require further investigations of the effects of these compounds on isolated CFTR channels in membrane patches as patch clamp assays.

4.2   Dynamic Selectivity

In view of previous reports that CFTR is permeable to HCO_3^- when activated by cAMP/ATP,[19-22] we were intrigued to find that when glutamate alone activated CFTR gCl$^-$, HCO_3^- remained impermeant and even more fascinated when after adding ATP in the presence of glutamate, HCO_3^- permeability returned to CFTR (Figure2, 4, 7).

4.2.1   Relative Magnitude

The actual ATP/glutamate activated HCO_3^- conductance varies somewhat from preparation to preparation.   It is noteworthy that relative to Cl$^-$, glutamate/ATP activated HCO_3^- conductance may exceed classically activated HCO_3^- conductance. These results may suggest that under more optimal conditions, CFTR gHCO$_3^-$ may increase even further. In any case, we believe this is the first demonstration of an anion channel dynamically changing its relative anionic selectivity in response to a cytosolic agent.

4.2.2   ATP Hydrolysis, Yes

Moreover, the change apparently requires the hydrolysis of ATP since it was not supported by the non-hydrolyzable ATP analogue, AMP-PNP (β−γ-imidoadenosine 5'-phosphate). This requirement indicates that CFTR must undergo an energy requiring structural transformation in order to assume permeability to HCO_3^-.

4.2.3   Phosphorylation, No

Like glutamate activation of CFTR gCl^-, activation of CFTR $gHCO_3^-$ apparently does not require kinase phosphorylation since stimulation of CFTR $gHCO_3^-$ survived kinase inhibition by staurosporine (Figure 6). We also note that the estimated Km (~2 mM) for ATP activation of $gHCO_3^-$ was significantly larger than the Km for ATP in most kinase mediated phosphorylation reactions.[23] Thus, if a kinase were phosphorylating CFTR to activate $gHCO_3^-$, $gHCO_3^-$ should have appeared when we added sub mM concentrations of ATP.

4.3   Evidence of CFTR Activation

4.3.1   Indirect Evidence

Given the novelty and complexity of the responses reported here for CFTR, it is more than tempting to assume that the responses may be due to the activity of more than one anion channel or at least in addition to CFTR. There are several indirect reasons, however, that protest that the conductances are those of CFTR: 1.) We have not found evidence of any other Cl^- channels on the apical membrane of the sweat duct.[24,25] 2.) The magnitude of the maximal gCl response to glutamate was approximately the same as for classical stimulation with cAMP/ATP (Figure 3). It would seem very unusual for two distant channels to exhibit the same conductance in the same tissue with independent activation. 3.) If another channel were involved, we would expect an increase in the total Cl^- conductance when we combined the agonists. However, adding ATP or ATP and cAMP together with glutamate did not increase the total gCl^- response over glutamate alone (Figure 3). The response was completely independent of Ca^{++} (unpublished observations).[24,25] Thus, it is not likely that a Ca^{++} activated Cl^- channel is involved. 5.) To our knowledge, CFTR is the only anion channel that can bind and hydrolyze ATP. The fact that hydrolyzable ATP is required to activate $gHCO_3^-$ in glutamate-stimulated channels suggests that the channel must interact with and hydrolyze this nucleotide. The strongest evidence that glutamate is activating CFTR and that ATP activates its HCO_3^- conductance derives from tissues where CFTR is known to be absent or defective.

4.3.2   Direct Evidence

ΔF508/ΔF508. We examined ducts from patients diagnosed with Cystic Fibrosis who were known to be homozygous for the ΔF508 mutation. This genotype is well characterized as a defect in protein processing that places little CFTR in the plasma membrane.[9]   When we applied glutamate or glutamate + ATP, we observed no detectable increase in either Cl⁻ or HCO_3^- conductances (Figure 11).   This finding firmly establishes that the conductance activation is dependent on functional CFTR, although it does not exclude the possibility that there may be some other anion channel that is completely dependent on the presence of CFTR. Even so, for the most part, the arguments above are difficult to reconcile with this alternative.

ΔF508/R117H. We then examined the response of tissue from patients heterozygous for mutations of the CF gene.   We considered the ΔF508 mutation to be mute, but R117H is known to result in Cl⁻ conductance increases that are significantly lower than WT (but not absent).[26]   We reasoned that if the glutamate activated conductances were through CFTR, there should be at least a partial increase in gCl⁻ and $gHCO_3^-$. While we are cautious about interpreting findings from a very limited number of experiments, the results not only appear to confirm that CFTR is the target of glutamate stimulation, but they suggest further insights into the pathology of the disease.

4.4   Implications for CF

We were impressed to find that $gHCO_3^-$ seems not to be seriously impaired by the R117H mutation. Despite the fact that the gCl⁻ response of R117H to glutamine appeared to be only about 15% of the response of WT, the $gHCO_3^-$ response to glutamate +ATP in R117H was almost 50% of WT. Superficially (we examined ducts from only two patients), these results suggest that the $gHCO_3^-$ function of the R117H mutation has little effect on $gHCO_3^-$, while it significantly depresses gCl⁻. These results are not without clinical correlation and support earlier observations in cells transfected with this mutation.[27]

Since defining the gene for Cystic Fibrosis,[28-30] it has been possible to establish some correlation between genotype and phenotypic expression. Perhaps the best-established correlation is with pancreatic function. That is, most patients (>95%) with cystic fibrosis mutations that are not functional (e.g., ΔF508, G551D, G542X) lose pancreatic function while mutations that appear to permit partial function remain pancreatic sufficient (R117H, R334W, P574H).[31-33] Taking these facts together with the fact that the organ of HCO_3^- transport is the pancreas presents an irrefutable message that CFTR is essential for HCO_3^- transport.

It is not surprising that we find no Cl^- or HCO_3^- conductance in $\Delta F508/\Delta F508$, since little if any CFTR protein is in the apical membrane.[34] Neither is it surprising that gCl^- is reduced in $\Delta F508/R117H$. But the fact that $gHCO_3^-$ is apparently much less affected than gCl^- in R117H is not only surprising, but offers excellent insight into why patients with this class of mutations are generally (70-80%) pancreatic sufficient.[31] The presence of pancreatic insufficiency among patients of this class of mutations may be explained and depend, at least in part, on the presence of different alleles associated with the gene. In this specific case, Cystic Fibrosis occurs with the $\Delta F508/R117H$ genotype if the T7 repeat allele in intron 8 occurs as a T5 repeat, which results in lower expression of the R117H gene.[35]

Presumably, if R117H appears in a normal T7 backgrounds, the $\Delta F508/R117H$ genotype would deliver approximately one half of the WT amount of protein to the membrane. If we assume that the sweat ducts from both CF patients with the $\Delta F508/R117H$ genotype examined here were of the T5 allele, we should also assume that less than one half the amount of CFTR normally expressed in WT will be present in the membrane. The fact that we see approximately 50% of the WT $gHCO_3^-$ in these ducts suggests that either: 1. The data overestimates the actual function or 2.) R117H mutations may even enhance $gHCO_3^-$. In any case, the fact that significant $gHCO_3^-$ escapes the R117H defect as shown here in the sweat duct indicates that it also escapes the defect in the pancreas, which very probably explains why most of these patients retain pancreatic function. Moreover, most patients that retain pancreatic function also fare better with lung pathology. This clinical result may suggest that the bicarbonate transport is critical to pulmonary defense, perhaps even more so than Cl^- transport. However, other potential roles should, perhaps, be considered.

4.5 Roles for Glutamate Activation of CFTR

The finding that glutamate and its precursors can activate CFTR without cAMP is puzzling. Currently, we do not know what role this activation serves in normal physiological function.

4.5.1 Energy Charge

It is known that α–keto glutarate, glutamate, and glutamine are intrinsically part of the energy reserves of the cell by virtue of their ability to enter the citric acid cycle and that they participate in feed back systems which stabilize cellular energy charge. Thus, at least, in absorptive epithelium such as the sweat duct, tying the functional status of CFTR to the cytoplasmic level of these intermediates may serve to keep CFTR tonically activated so long as there is sufficient energy available to support the demands of transcellular salt transport. It will be intriguing to see whether the same phenomenon exists in secretory cells, where the secretory function cannot be maintained tonically activated. (In absorption, the fluid substrate for absorption is provided by prior isotonic fluid secretion; thus, absorptive activity is an obligate slave of secretion, and even though CFTR is tonically open, no absorption can occur unless sweat secretion precedes it.)

4.5.2   Volume Regulation

Glutamate may participate as a regulated osmolyte in the control of cell volume.[12,36] Influx and efflux of salt can also cause wide fluctuations in epithelial cell volume.[37] We might speculate then that an increase in cell volume, which would follow loading the cell with Cl^- when CFTR is open, would lower cell glutamate (and/or precursor) concentrations favoring lower CFTR activity and lower gCl^-, thus lowering Cl^- uptake to assist a return to normal volume. This function would seem to require a very steep dependence on glutamate concentration.

4.5.3   pH and HCO_3^- Conductance

While the above speculation may have some rationale in terms of known physiological demands, it seems much more difficult to place the ATP dependent dynamic change in CFTR HCO_3^- selectivity in a physiological role. Since HCO_3^- is a major intracellular buffer and the most important extracellular buffer, this dynamic regulation of CFTR seems most likely to be related to some function of intracellular pH regulation and, of course, HCO_3^- transport. Such involvement is suggested all the more by the fact that glutamine is central to pH regulation in the kidney and probably other tissues.[38,39]

5.   CONCLUSIONS

Using the basolaterally permeabilized, microperfused native human sweat duct, we have discovered that CFTR in the apical membrane can be activated by the exogenous addition of low mM levels of three distinct 5 carbon chain carboxylic acids: α-keto glutarate, glutamate, and glutamine. Activation of CFTR by these substances alone induces a Cl^- permeable, HCO_3^- impermeable state in this tissue that is comparable in magnitude to that elicited by classical activation with cAMP and ATP via protein kinase A phosphorylation. Including mM levels of ATP with these substances appears to induce or to allow a change of state in CFTR that is permeable to both Cl⁻ and HCO_3^-. Thus, we find the first evidence of an induced dynamic change in ion selectivity of an active anion channel. This novel activation appears to be independent of phosphorylation, but the change in selectivity appears to be dependent on ATP hydrolysis. Evidence that these responses are properties of CFTR is derived from tissues from cystic fibrosis patients that show CFTR mutation (genotype) specific responses. The physiological role of glutamate activation remains to be defined, but we speculate that it may involve controls of cellular energy charge, cell volume, and/or intracellular pH.

ACKNOWLEDGMENTS

NIH DK51899-01, NIH DE14352, and the Olmsted Trust supported this work. We express deep appreciation for the technical assistance of Ms. Suchi Maddireddi, BS and Mr. Kirk Taylor, MS.

REFERENCES

1. M. M. Reddy and P. M. Quinton. cAMP activation of CF-affected Cl- conductance in both cell membranes of an absorptive epithelium. *J. Membr. Biol.* **130**, 49-62 (1992).
2. K. Sato and F. Sato. Defective beta adrenergic response of cystic fibrosis sweat glands in vivo and in vitro. *J. Clin. Invest.* **73**, 1763-71 (1984).
3. J. Bijman and P. Quinton. Permeability properties of cell membranes and tight junctions of normal and cystic fibrosis sweat ducts. *Pflugers Arch.* **408**, 505-10 (1987).
4. R. Greger. Cation selectivity of the isolated perfused cortical thick ascending limb of Henle's loop of rabbit kidney. *Pflugers Arch.* **390**, 30-7 (1981).
5. M. M. Reddy and P. M. Quinton. Intracellular potentials of microperfused human sweat duct cells. *Pflugers Arch.* **410**, 471-5 (1987).
6. P. M. Quinton and M. M. Reddy. Cl⁻ conductance and acid secretion in the human sweat duct. *Ann. N. Y. Acad. Sci.* **574**, 438-46 (1989).
7. P. M. Quinton and M. M. Reddy. Control of CFTR chloride conductance by ATP levels through non-hydrolytic binding. *Nature* **360**, 79-81 (1992).
8. T. Tamaoki and H. Nakano. Potent and specific inhibitors of protein kinase C of microbial origin. *Biotechnology (N Y)* **8**, 732-5 (1990).
9. S. H. Cheng, et al. Defective intracellular transport and processing of CFTR is the molecular basis of most cystic fibrosis. *Cell* **63**, 827-34 (1990).
10. M. M. Reddy and P. M. Quinton. Control of dynamic CFTR selectivity by glutamate and ATP in epithelial cells. *Nature* **423**, 756 - 760 (2003).
11. Y. Kera, et al. Presence of free D-glutamate and D-aspartate in rat tissues. *Biochim. Biophys. Acta* **1243**, 283-6 (1995).

12. V. Dall'Asta, et al. Amino acids are compatible osmolytes for volume recovery after hypertonic shrinkage in vascular endothelial cells. *Am. J. Physiol.* **276**, C865-72 (1999).

13. R. Fussle, et al. On the mechanism of membrane damage by Staphylococcus aureus alphatoxin. *J. Cell Biol.* **91**, 83-94 (1981).

14. C. L. Bell and P. M. Quinton. Regulation of CFTR Cl⁻ conductance in secretion by cellular energy levels. *Am. J. Physiol.* **264**, C925-31 (1993).

15. D. A. Flockhart, W. Freist, J. Hoppe, T. M. Lincoln and J. D. Corbin. ATP analog specificity of cAMP-dependent protein kinase, cGMP-dependent protein kinase, and phosphorylase kinase. *Eur. J. Biochem.* **140**, 289-95 (1984).

16. W. R. Taylor and N. M. Green. The predicted secondary structures of the nucleotide-binding sites of six cation-transporting ATPases lead to a probable tertiary fold. *Eur. J. Biochem.* **179**, 241-8 (1989).

17. P. M. Quinton and M. M. Reddy. Regulation of absorption in the human sweat duct. *Adv. Exp. Med. Biol.* **290**, 159-70; discussion 170-2 (1991).

18. P. M. Quinton and M. M. Reddy. Regulation of absorption by phosphorylation of CFTR. *Jpn. J. Physiol.* **44** Suppl 2, S207-13 (1994).

19. J. A. Tabcharani and J. W. Hanrahan. Permeation in the cystic fibrosis transmembrane conductance regulator (CFTR) chloride channel. *Biophys .J.* **64**, A17 (1993).

20. J. H. Poulsen, H. Fischer, B. Illek and T. E. Machen. Bicarbonate conductance and pH regulatory capability of cystic fibrosis transmembrane conductance regulator. *Proc. Natl. Acad. Sci. U. S. A.* **91**, 5340-4 (1994).

21. B. Illek, A. W. Tam, H. Fischer, and T. E. Machen. Anion selectivity of apical membrane conductance of Calu 3 human airway epithelium. *Pflugers Arch.* **437**, 812-22 (1999).

22. P. M. Quinton and M. M. Reddy. CFTR, a rectifying, non-rectifying anion channel? *J. Korean Med. Sci.* **15** Suppl, S17-20 (2000).

23. M. P. Anderson, et al. Nucleoside triphosphates are required to open the CFTR chloride channel. *Cell* **67**, 775-84 (1991).

24. M. M. Reddy and P. M. Quinton. Rapid regulation of electrolyte absorption in sweat duct. *J. Membr. Biol.* **140**, 57-67 (1994).

25. M. M. Reddy and P. M. Quinton. Deactivation of CFTR-Cl conductance by endogenous phosphatases in the native sweat duct. *Am. J. Physiol.* **270**, C474-80 (1996).

26. D. N. Sheppard, et al. Mutations in CFTR associated with mild-disease-form Cl- channels with altered pore properties. *Nature* **362**, 160-4 (1993).

27. J. Y. Choi, et al. Aberrant CFTR-dependent HCO₃⁻ transport in mutations associated with cystic fibrosis. *Nature* **410**, 94-7 (2001).

28. B. Kerem, et al. Identification of the cystic fibrosis gene: genetic analysis. *Science* **245**, 1073-80 (1989).

29. J. R. Riordan, et al. Identification of the cystic fibrosis gene: cloning and characterization of complementary DNA. *Science* **245**, 1066-73 (1989).

30. J. M. Rommens, et al. Identification of the cystic fibrosis gene: chromosome walking and jumping. *Science* **245**, 1059-65 (1989).

31. P. Kristidis, et al. Genetic determination of exocrine pancreatic function in cystic fibrosis. *Am. J. Hum. Genet.* **50**, 1178-84 (1992).

32. C. Durno, et al. Genotype and phenotype correlations in patients with cystic fibrosis and pancreatitis. *Gastroenterology* **123**, 1857-64 (2002).

33. R. K. Rowntree and A. Harris. The phenotypic consequences of CFTR mutations. *Ann. Hum. Genet.* **67**, 471-85 (2003).

34. N. Kartner, O. Augustinas, T. J. Jensen, A. L. Naismith, and J. R. Riordan. Mislocalization of delta F508 CFTR in cystic fibrosis sweat gland. *Nat. Genet.* **1**, 321-7 (1992).

35. S. Kiesewetter, et al. A mutation in CFTR produces different phenotypes depending on chromosomal background. *Nat. Genet.* **5**, 274-8 (1993).

36. N. MacAulay, U. Gether, D. A. Klaerke and T. Zeuthen. Water transport by the human Na$^+$-coupled glutamate cotransporter expressed in Xenopus oocytes. *J. Physiol.* **530**, 367-78 (2001).

37. L. Reuss. Cell volume regulation in nonrenal epithelia. *Renal Physiology and Biochemistry* **3-5**, 187-201 (1988).

38. N. P. Curthoys and M. Watford. Regulation of glutaminase activity and glutamine metabolism. *Annu. Rev. Nutr.* **15**, 133-59 (1995).

39. I. Nissim. Newer aspects of glutamine/glutamate metabolism: the role of acute pH changes. *Am. J. Physiol.* **277**, F493-7 (1999).

Chapter 2

ROLE OF CFTR AND OTHER ION CHANNELS IN CYSTIC FIBROSIS

Karl Kunzelmann[1], Tanja Bachhuber[1], Gabriele Adam[1], Thilo Voelcker[1], Bettina Mürle[1], Marcus Mall[2], and Rainer Schreiber[1]

[1]*Institut für Physiologie, Universität Regensburg, Universitätstraße 31, D-93053 Regensburg, Germany. Tel: +49 (0) 941 943 4302, Fax: +49 (0) 941 943 4315, uqkkunze@mailbox.uq.edu.au.* [2]*Cystic Fibrosis/Pulmonary Research and Treatment Center, School of Medicine. The University of North Carolina at Chapel Hill. 7011 Thurston Bowles Building, Chapel Hill, NC 27599-7248, USA.*

1. INTRODUCTION

Cystic fibrosis is the most common severe inherited disease among the Caucasian population. It is caused by mutations in the CFTR (cystic fibrosis transmembrane conductance regulator) protein, a Cl^- channel that plays a central role in the process of ion secretion and absorption in epithelial tissues. CFTR is expressed in polarized epithelial cells together with a number of other channels, carriers and pumps. Mutations in the CFTR gene lead to a defect in Cl^- secretion in these epithelial tissues. This has been proposed to be the cause for clinical symptoms observed in cystic fibrosis.[1,2] However, some of the transport defects observed in *in vivo* measurements in cystic fibrosis patients, in tissues from CF patients, or in transgenic mice, carrying CFTR mutations, cannot be reconciled with the concept of a defective Cl^- conductance as the single resaon for the transport defects observed in CF (Figure 1).[2-4] Because CFTR is regulated by second messengers, cytosolic factors and membrane receptors[5] and also regulates other membrane conductances, epithelial transport properties are largely dependent on CFTR function (Figure 1). In this short review, we will discuss the role of CFTR during secretion and absorption of electrolytes and will elucidate the contribution of basolateral K^+ channels to epithelial transport.

We will then describe the correlation between the epithelial Na⁺ channel ENaC, CFTR and stimulation by purinergic agonists. New aspects of pharmacotherapy of cystic fibrosis and pharmacological manipulation of ion channel activity will be reviewed. Thus, this review will focus on the role of CFTR in the airway epithelium.

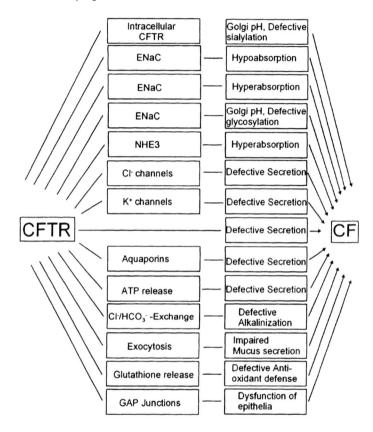

Figure 1. Summary of the effects of CFTR on membrane transport proteins in vitro and in vivo and putative impact on pathophysiology and phenotype in cystic fibrosis.

2.   CFTR, CYSTIC FIBROSIS AND DEFECTIVE EPITHELIAL ION TRANSPORT

The CFTR protein is located in both secretory as well as absorptive epithelial cells. In the airways, CFTR is located predominantly in the luminal membrane of cells forming serous end pieces of submucosal glands (Figure 2). Thus, most Cl⁻ secretion takes place in the serous part of the submucosal glands and is in charge of flushing the submucosal glands, thereby removing mucus (Figure 2). It is easily conceivable that a defect in CFTR mediated Cl⁻ secretion will lead to accumulation of mucus within the glands, occlusion of the ducts and inflammation. Apart from expression of CFTR in the submucosal glands, expression is also found in the superficial epithelium, although to a lesser degree. Here, CFTR is forming an absorptive pathway for Cl⁻ ions, similar to the function of CFTR in the sweat duct. As shown in Figure 3, ion transport in either secretory or absorptive direction requires additional transport proteins. Thus, Cl⁻ secretion requires accumulation of Cl⁻ inside the cell by the basolateral $Na^+/2Cl^-/K^+$-cotransporter (NKCC1). Basolateral K^+ channels serve as a recycling mechanism for K^+ ions and hyperpolarize the cell membranes, which facilitates and maintains electrolyte secreting. The basolateral shunt pathway allows secretion of Na^+ to the luminal side, which is driven by the lumen negative transepithelial voltage. In the absorptive superficial epithelium, CFTR colocalizes with epithelial Na^+ channels (ENaC) and due to the depolarizing effect of Na^+ absorption, Cl⁻ is driven in the absorptive direction. Cl⁻ ions are released to the basolateral compartment via anion exchangers, KCl cotransporter or basolaterally located Cl⁻ channels. As indicated for the Cl⁻ secretion, absorption of Cl⁻ ions does require a basolateral K^+ conductance. The molecular nature of these basolateral K^+ channels will be discussed in the next chapter. Ultimately, both secretion and absorption are driven by the ATP consuming Na^+/K^+ - ATPase.

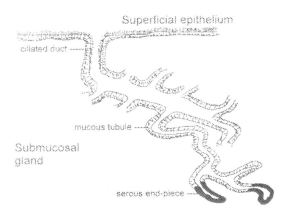

Figure 2. Model of a submucosal gland in human airways.

Cystic fibrosis is characterized by inadequate ion secretion in conjunction with enhanced NaCl absorption in airways and colon. Hypoabsorption of NaCl has been observed for other tissues such as the sweat duct epithelium.

This leads to the well described phenomenon of enhanced salt excretion with the sweat.[6] However, apart from this and the gastrointestinal symptoms observed in CF, the progressive lung disease is the single most important and life limiting factor in CF. According to the so called isotonic volume hypothesis[7], at least two mechanisms contribute to the CF lung disease: i) enhanced absorption of Na^+, and consequently, hyperabsorption of fluid and electrolytes by the airway surface epithelium, and ii) impaired cAMP dependent Cl^- secretion. Both transport defects have been detected initially in short circuit measurements in excised CF airways and cultured CF airway epithelial cells.[3,8] Patch clamp analysis on CF airway epithelial cells identified enhanced amiloride sensitive whole cell currents and an increase in the activity of the Na^+ channel.[9,10] These results are confirmed by microelectrode measurements and Ussing chamber recordings on freshly isolated CF respiratory tissues.[10] Moreover, the nasal potential difference (PD) *in vivo* in CF patients showed enhanced amiloride induced PD changes and hyperabsorption of Na^+ along with defective Cl^- secretion. The so called isotonic volume transport theory[7,11] predicts an isotonic contraction of the airway surface liquid (ASL), the thin watery layer that covers the ciliated airway epithelial cells. Dehydration of the ASL leads to impaired mucociliary clearance as a key factor in innate lung defense, and results in mucus impactions on airway surfaces. In contrast, an alternative low salt or defensin theory predicts a low salt or hypotonic ASL under normal conditions, and an increase in ASL tonicity in CF airways. Accordingly, it has been proposed that hypertonic ASL inhibits the activity of antimicrobial defensin like molecules.[12,13] However, subsequent measurements of the salt

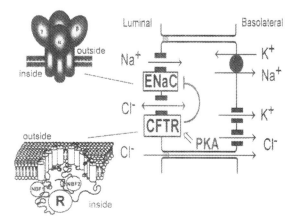

Figure 3. Model for regulation of epithelial Na^+ channels (ENaC) by CFTR. In airway epithelial cells.

concentration and properties of the ASL using more sophisticated methods did not reveal an increased salt concentration in the ASL of CF patients.[14-16] While an increase in ASL tonicity is unlikely to occur in CF, airway mucus accumulation, occlusion of small airways and a defective HCO_3^- secretion are very likely to be major determinants of the CF airway disease.[17,18]

3.   CONTRIBUTION OF BASOLATERAL POTASSIUM CHANNELS IN EPITHELIA

Basolateral K^+ channels are essential to maintain a hyperpolarized membrane voltage and the electrical driving force that is required for Cl^- secretion and Na^+ absorption (Figure 4). Similar to intestinal epithelia, also airways posses at least two different types of K^+ channels, which are activated either by increases in intracellular Ca^{2+} or camp/[19,20] Ca^{2+} activated K^+ channels maintain the negative membrane voltage in resting epithelial cells and supply the driving force during Ca^{2+} mediated stimulation of secretion.[21] However, when intracellular cAMP is enhanced and luminal Cl^- channels are activated, the cells depolarize. Under these conditions, Ca^{2+} influx into the cell is limited and Ca^{2+} dependent K^+ channels become less active.[22-24] Loss of activity of Ca^{2+} activated K^+ channels is compensated by parallel activation of cAMP dependent K^+ channels, repolarizing the membrane voltage.[25] Apart from these two types of K^+ channels, other K^+ conductances may also participate in maintaining the negative membrane voltage, but are currently only poorly characterized.[26,27] Thus, it is not clear to what degree a large conductance Ca^{2+} dependent K^+ channel contributes to the basolateral K^+ conductance in airway epithelial cells. The cAMP activated K^+ conductance can be blocked specifically by the chromanol compound 293B.[20,28] The channel was initially cloned from heart muscle and was named K_VLQT1 (KCNQ1), indicating its role in the long QT-syndrome. K_VLQT1 is the α subunit in a K^+ channel complex together with the small regulatory β subunit, KCNE3.[20,29,30] KCNE3 has a large impact on K^+ channel properties and pharmacology, similar to those of minK (KCNE1, IsK).[29,31,32]

The open probability of the Ca^{2+} activated K^+ channel is largely enhanced by increase in intracellular Ca^{2+}.[22,33,34] Moreover, evidence exists that the channel activity is modulated by phosphorylation.[24] This channel has been isolated initially from human brain cells (hSK4), pancreas (hIK1) and T cells (hKCa4; KCNN4).[35-38] The channel is also activated by 1-ethyl-2-benzimidazolone (1-EBIO).[39-42] Patch clamp studies showed that the channel is blocked by low concentrations of the antifungal antibiotic clotrimazole and the imidazole compounds clotrimazole.[41]

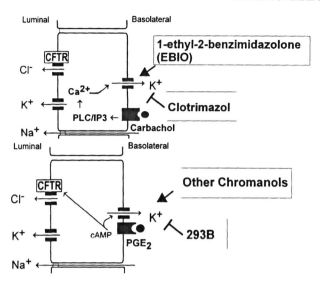

Figure 4. Model of secretion by airway epithelial cells. Contribution of basolateral K^+ channels activated by increase of intracellular Ca^{2+} (upper model) or cAMP (lower model).

4. INHIBITION OF THE EPITHELIAL SODIUM CHANNEL ENAC BY CFTR

Regulation of the epithelial Na^+ channel ENaC by CFTR Cl^- channels was first detected in an epithelial cell line and in fibroblasts transfected with ENaC and CFTR.[43] Amiloride sensitive short circuit currents, as detected in Ussing chamber recordings, and amiloride sensitive whole cell currents were found to be inhibited by cAMP in cells co-transfected with CFTR. These initial results were confirmed by a subsequent study, in which CFTR and ENaC were coexpressed in oocytes of *Xenopus laevis*. Amiloride sensitive whole cell currents were measured using the double electrode voltage clamp method.[44] ENaC currents were inhibited by activation of wtCFTR Cl^- currents, but not by mutant ΔF508-CFTR. Several subsequent studies used basically identical techniques and arrived at similar conclusions. Notably, a CFTR inhibition of amiloride sensitive Na^+ absorption was observed in Ussing chamber studies on both human airways and colon. This inhibition was not seen in tissues from CF patients.[10,45] Moreover, Ussing chamber studies on the mouse colon revealed cAMP dependent inhibition of amiloride sensitive short circuit currents in normal, but not in transgenic G551D-CFTR mice.[46] These results were further supported by other techniques such as microelectrodes and whole cell patch clamp recordings, which were applied to native human and rat epithelial cells.[10,47] Finally, the open probability (Po) of ENaC channels reconstituted into planar lipid bilayers was determined and a decrease in the single channel Po was found by activation of co-reconstituted CFTR.[48] The results from the different studies suggest a twofold effect of CFTR on amiloride sensitive transport: i) The baseline Na$^+$ conductance in the non-stimulated tissue is reduced without activation of CFTR. ii) After stimulation of wtCFTR by cAMP, amiloride sensitive Na$^+$ absorption is further inhibited. The situation is very different in the sweat duct, where activation of CFTR does not inhibit but increases Na$^+$ absorption.[6,49] Accordingly, the defect in NaCl absorption in the CF sweat duct is due to both defective Na$^+$ and Cl$^-$ channel function. The reason for the different impact of CFTR on ENaC in airways and sweat duct remains obscure. Numerous studies have shown a decrease of ENaC currents during activation of CFTR in *Xenopus* oocytes.[44,50-54] CFTR's ability to downregulate ENaC largely depends on the direction and the magnitude of the Cl$^-$ current through CFTR Cl$^-$ channels.[55] Thus, Cl$^-$ flux through CFTR and/or changes in the intracellular Cl$^-$ concentration could serve as the signal for inhibition of ENaC (Figure 5). The inhibitory effects of CFTR on ENaC are clearly suppressed in the presence of a low extracellular Cl$^-$ concentration, suggesting that Cl$^-$ influx and eventually accumulation in the cytosol is essential for the inhibition of EnaC.[52,55] Such a mechanism exists in the mouse salivary duct epithelium.[56,57] For this feedback regulation of ENaC, G$_{\alpha i2}$ subunits of Cl$^-$ sensitive trimeric GTP binding proteins play a central role. However, recent experiments exclude a role of G proteins in the downregulation of ENaC by CFTR in *Xenopus* oocytes.[53]

The results challenge the question whether Cl$^-$ currents generated by other Cl$^-$ channels, are also able to inhibit ENaC. In fact, inhibition of ENaC is not unique to CFTR, but is also caused by other Cl$^-$ conductances and consecutive increase in the intracellular Cl$^-$ concentration. Thus, ENaC is inhibited in amphotericin B permeabilized oocytes by increasing the bath Cl$^-$ concentration from 5 to 50 mmol/l.[52] Furthermore, another type of Cl$^-$ channel, the ClC-0 channel, was coexpressed together with ENaC which also inhibited EnaC.[52] This result has been confirmed recently by experiments coexpressing CFTR with ClC-2 Cl$^-$ channels.[58]The question is, after all, how do Cl$^-$ ions actually inhibit ENaC? This is currently under examination, yet, preliminary experiments suggest a direct interference of Cl$^-$ ions with the ENaC channel. Previous experiments in *Xenopus* oocytes excluded the contribution of Cl$^-$ sensitive proteins, such as GTP binding proteins and the nucleoside diphosphate kinase (NDPK).[51,53] A current working hypothesis proposes a model in which Cl$^-$ ions interfere with positive charges, located in close proximity to the inner mouth of ENaC channels, thereby inhibiting

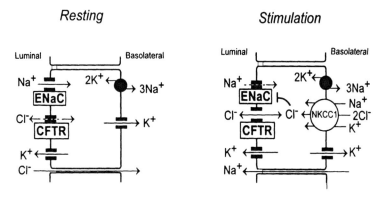

Figure 5. Epithelial cells under resting conditions and after stimulation with secretagogues.

permeation of Na⁺ ions through EnaC.[59] In good agreement with such a model are results from recent patch clamp experiments which show reduced Na⁺ channel currents in the presence of a high cytosolic Cl⁻ concentration.[59] Using different techniques such as Western blots, double electrode voltage clamp and patch clamp experiments, binding sides for phosphatidylinositol 4,5-bisphosphate (PIP$_2$) have been identified in the N termini of β,γ-ENaC.[60,61] Negatively charged PIP$_2$ regulates ENaC at the level of the inner plasma membrane through a mechanism that is independent of ENaC trafficking. It remains to be shown, whether a similar scenario applies to the CFTR mediated inhibition of ENaC.

How do the results obtained in *Xenopus* oocytes compare to the situation in epithelial tissues? Apart from a few early studies on the intracellular Na⁺ and Cl⁻ concentration in airway epithelial cells, not much is known about changes in the intracellular Cl⁻ concentration during acute stimulation of airway and colonic epithelial cells.[62-66] Possibly only the Cl⁻ concentration close to the cell membrane and in close proximity to ENaC may be relevant for Na⁺ channel inhibition. Opening of luminal Cl⁻ channels may increase cellular uptake and absorption of both Cl⁻ and Na⁺ and thereby inhibit ENaC. Increase in intracellular Cl⁻ activity may occur initially by an influx of Cl⁻ through apically located CFTR Cl⁻ channels. However, secretagogues also activate the basolateral Na⁺/2Cl⁻/K⁺ cotransporter (NKCC1), which leads to an uptake of Cl⁻ into the cell. Recent experiments were performed in our laboratory on mouse kidney collecting duct cells, which have been transfected with a construct expressing the Cl⁻ sensitive yellow fluorescent protein YFP. M1 cells express ENaC along with CFTR and NKCC1 and exhibit quenching of the fluorescence during activation of CFTR by secretagogues.[67-69] This indicated an increase in [Cl⁻]$_i$ concentration by about 17 mmol/l. Replacing the extracellular Ringer solution by a low (5 mmol/l)

Cl⁻ solution induced an efflux of Cl⁻ and a dequenching of the fluorescence signal. The efflux was more pronounced, and thus the slope of the fluorescence increase was steeper after stimulation of additional CFTR Cl⁻ channels (Figure 6). These data demonstrate that stimulation of M1 cells and thus activation of CFTR Cl⁻ channels causes an uptake of Cl⁻ and increase in $[Cl^-]_i$.

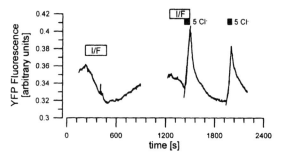

Figure 6. Change of YFP fluorescence in mouse collecting duct cells upon stimulation with IBMX and forskolin and in the presence of high (145 mmol/l) or low (5 mmol/l) extracellular Cl⁻ concentration.

5.   PURINERGIC REGULATION OF ENAC AND CL⁻ CONDUCTANCE

Activation of electrolyte secretion by stimulation with extracellular nucleotides in both normal and CF airways is well described.[70-73] It has been demonstrated that basolateral application of ATP to human airway epithelial cells activates Cl⁻ secretion indirectly, by activating K⁺ channels, while luminal application of ATP and UTP activates alternative Ca^{2+}-dependent Cl⁻ channels, in murine and human normal and CF respiratory epithelia via binding to purinergic $P2Y_2$ receptors.[19,71,74-77] $P2Y_2$ receptors couple to intracellular protein lipase C (PLC) and G-proteins, and thereby increase intracellular Ca^{2+} upon activation.[74,78] $P2Y_2$ receptors are co-localized with $P2Y_6$ and probably $P2Y_4$ receptors on the mucosal side of the epithelium.[79-82] The luminal $P2Y_2$ receptor is activated by ATP or UTP, while $P2Y_6$ receptors are stimulated through metabolic break down products of UTP, such as UDP.[83] ATP and UTP are released constitutively and in response to mechanical stress *in vitro* and *in vivo* during coughing.[84,85] ATP release has been demonstrated to be CFTR independent and to occur during membrane stretch.[80,86] Luminal ATP/UTP activates Ca^{2+} dependent Cl⁻ channels of unknown molecular identity.[87-89] A family of apparently Ca^{2+} / calmodulin activated Cl⁻ channels (hCaCC-1, hCaCC-2, hCaCC-3) have been found to be expressed in the digestive and respiratory mucosa and are thus candidate proteins for the luminal Ca^{2+} activated Cl^- channel.[19,90,91] The recently identified family of bestrophins are other potential candidates.[92,93] As mentioned above, activation of luminal Cl^- channels is paralleled by activation of basolateral Ca^{2+} dependent K^+ channels.[19,94]

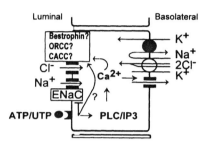

Figure 7. Regulation of ion transport by purinergic stimulation.

Activation of mucosal purinergic receptors does not only stimulate Cl^- secretion but also modulates Na^+ absorption. This has been shown meanwhile for various epithelia, including kidney and airway epithelial cells.[77,95-97] In lung epithelia, inhibition of Na^+ transport by extracellular nucleotides has been reported for human and rabbit trachea, rat distal airway cells, porcine bronchi and cultured human bronchial epithelial cells.[77,95,98-100] In native human airway tissues, the fractional inhibition of the amiloride sensitive Na^+ transport was similar in normal and CF tissues.[77] However, due to enhanced basal Na^+ transport in CF, the absolute magnitude of nucleotide-mediated inhibition of Na^+ absorption is significantly increased in CF compared to normal tissues.[77] Although several transport proteins participate in transepithelial Na^+ absorption, such as luminal epithelial Na^+ channels (ENaC), the basolateral Na^+/K^+ ATPase and basolateral K^+ channels,[46] it is likely that purinergic stimulation inhibits ENaC directly.[60,101] The mechanism of ATP or UTP mediated inhibition of Na^+ absorption is currently under investigation. Ca^{2+} itself or Ca^{2+} dependent protein kinase C (PKC) are not in charge of the inhibition of amiloride sensitive Na^+ transport in the airways.[77,78] It has been shown that amiloride sensitive transport is inhibited by a G protein sensitive mechanism, that it requires the function of phospholipase C and also involves Cl^- transport over the luminal membrane.[78] Recent papers show activation of ENaC channels by phosphatidylinositols, probably by interaction with putative PIP_2 binding domains in the N-termini of the β and γ subunits of heterotetrameric ENaC channels. Hydrolysis of PIP_2 by phospholipase C to produce 1,4,5-inositol trisphosphate (IP_3) and diacylglycerol (DAG) leads to deactivation of ENaC channels.[60,61] Thus anionic phospholipids like PIP_2, abundantly present in the inner leaflet of eukaryotic plasma membranes, are not just precursors for intracellular second messengers but are in itself regulatory molecules.[102] According to this, cleavage of PIP_2 by activation of PLC through stimulation of purinergic receptors is probably the mechanism by which ENaC and thus amiloride sensitive Na^+ absorption is inhibited.[101]

6.   ION CHANNEL THERAPY IN CYSTIC FIBROSIS

Because defective Cl^- secretion and enhanced Na^+ absorption are crucial to the pathophysiology of the CF lung disease, normalizing the transport abnormalities are the major therapeutical target. Several strategies have been developed to overcome the reduced Cl^- secretion caused by defective CFTR Cl^- channel function. Accordingly, strategies aim at correcting the maturation and activity of mutant CFTR. These strategies have been outlined in previous reports.[103,104] As an alternative approach, transepithelial electrolyte secretion may be promoted by enhancing the driving force for luminal Cl^- exit. This can be achieved by activation of K^+ channels located on the basolateral side of the epithelium. While activators for the cAMP regulated KCNQ1 K^+ channel are not yet readily available, specific openers for the Ca^{2+} activated K^+ channel have been identified meanwhile. Among these, the benzimidazolone compounds 1-EBIO or chlorzoxazone have been found to hyperpolarize the basolateral membrane of epithelial cells (Figure 4).[40,105] Other efforts focus on inhibition of epithelial Na^+ channels to counteract the enhanced Na^+ absorption.[106] Early clinical trials using aerosolized amiloride showed some improvement in mucociliary clearance in the airways of CF patients.[107,108] The limited evidence for a positive long-term benefit[109,110] may be due to the rapid clearance of amiloride from the airways.

As outlined above, topical application of aerosolized ATP or UTP could have a dual therapeutic effect by counteracting increased Na^+ absorption and promoting Ca^{2+} dependent Cl^- secretion in airways from CF patients. *In vivo*, however, both UTP and ATP are rapidly degraded (< 1 min) from the airways by ecto-nucleotidases, limiting the therapeutic effects of both nucleotides. Thus, efforts are put into the development of more stable and longer lasting ligands of purinergic receptors. In that respect, it has been suggested to combine stable analogues of UTP with long acting Na^+ channel blockers, such as loperamide.[111] Recently, synthetic ligands of purinergic receptors have been developed, with a higher biological and chemical stability compared to UTP or ATP.[112-114] Novel $P2Y_2$ receptor agonist were developed for the treatment of CF. Initial results from clinical studies in normal volunteers demonstrate the safety of these compounds.[115] Recent, randomized, double-blinded, phase I studies with patients suffering from mild to moderate cystic fibrosis show promising results.[116] Thus, synthetic ligands of purinergic P2Y$_2$ receptors have a potential for future use in the treatment of cystic fibrosis.

ACKNOWLEDGEMENTS

This work was supported by NHMRC 252823 and ARC A00104609, the Else Kröner-Fresenius Stiftung. The excellent technical assistance by Ms. Ernestine Tartler and Ms. Agnes Paech is gratefully acknowledged. We thank Prof. Alan Verkman and Dr. Ma for providing us with the YFP constructs and Prof. Dr. C. Korbmacher for supplying the M1 cells.

REFERENCES

1. J. M. Pilewski and R. A. Frizzell, Role of CFTR in airway disease, *Physiol. Rev.* **79**, S215-S255 (1999).
2. K. Kunzelmann, The Cystic Fibrosis Transmembrane Conductance Regulator and its function in epithelial transport, *Rev. Physiol. Biochem. Pharmacol.* **137**, 1-70 (1999).
3. R. C. Boucher, C. U. Cotton, J. T. Gatzy, M. R. Knowles and J. R. Yankaskas, Evidence for reduced Cl$^-$ and increased Na$^+$ permeability in cystic fibrosis human primary cell cultures. *J. Physiol. (Lond)* **405**, 77-103 (1988).
4. B. R. Grubb and R. C. Boucher, Pathophysiology of gene-targeted mouse models for cystic fibrosis, *Physiol. Rev.* **79**, S193-S214 (1999).
5. K. Kunzelmann, Control of membrane transport by the cystic fibrosis transmembrane conductance regulator (CFTR). In K. L. Kirk and D. C. Dawson, eds., *The Cystic Fibrosis Transmembrane Conductance Regulator*, Landes Bioscience USA (in press) (2003).
6. M. M. Reddy and P. M. Quinton, Activation of the epithelial Na$^+$ channel (ENaC) requires CFTR Cl$^-$ channel function, *Nature* **402**, 301-304 (1999).
7. R. C. Boucher, Molecular insights into the physiology of the 'thin film' of airway surface liquid. *J. Physiol.* **516**, 631-638 (1999).
8. M. R. Knowles, M. J. Stutts, A. Spock, N. Fischer, J. T. Gatzy and R. C. Boucher, Abnormal Ion Permeation Though Cystic Fibrosis Respiratory Epithelium, *Science* **221**, 1067-1070 (1983).
9. T. C. Chinet, J. M. Fullton, J. R. Yankaskas, R. C. Boucher and M. J. Stutts, Mechanism of sodium hyperabsorbtion in cultured cystic fibrosis nasal epithelium: a patch clamp study, *Am. J. Physiol.* **266**, C1061-C1068 (1994).
10. M. Mall, M. Bleich, R. Greger, R. Schreiber and K. Kunzelmann, The amiloride inhibitable Na$^+$ conductance is reduced by CFTR in normal but not in CF airways, *J. Clin. Invest.* **102**, 15-21 (1998).

11. H. Matsui, C. W. Davis, R. Tarran and R. C. Boucher, Osmotic water permeabilities of cultured, well-differentiated normal and cystic fibrosis airway epithelia. *J. Clin. Invest.* **105**, 1419-1427 (2000).

12. J. Zabner, J. J. Smith, P. H. Karp, J. H. Widdicombe and M. J. Welsh, Loss of CFTR chloride channels alters salt absorption by cystic fibrosis airway epithelia in vitro, *Mol. Cell* **2**, 397-403 (1998).

13. P. M. Quinton, Viscosity versus composition in airway pathology, *Am. J. Respir. Crit. Care Med.* **149**, 6-7 (1994).

14. R. A. Caldwell, B. R. Grubb, R. Tarran, R. C. Boucher, M. R. Knowles and P. M. Barker, In Vivo Airway Surface Liquid Cl⁻ Analysis with Solid-state Electrodes, *J. Gen. Physiol.* **119**, 3-14 (2002).

15. R. Tarran, B. R. Grubb, D. Parsons, M. Picher, A. J. Hirsh, C. W. Davis and R. C. Boucher, The CF salt controversy: in vivo observations and therapeutic approaches, *Mol. Cell* **8**, 149-158 (2001).

16. S. Jayaraman, Y. Song and A. S. Verkman, Airway Surface Liquid Osmolality Measured using Fluorophore-encapsulated Liposomes, *J. Gen. Physiol.* **117**, 423-430 (2001).

17. J. H. Widdicombe, Regulation of the depth and composition of airway surface liquid, *J. Anat.* **201**, 313-318 (2002).

18. P. M. Quinton, The neglected ion: HCO_3^-, *Nat. Med.* **7**, 292-293 (2001).

19. M. Mall, T. Gonska, J. Thomas, R. Schreiber, H. H. Seydewitz, J. Kuehr, M. Brandis and K. Kunzelmann, Role of basolateral K⁺ channels in Ca^{2+} activated Cl⁻ secretion in human normal and cystic fibrosis airway epithelia, *Pediatric Research* **53**, 608-618 (2003).

20. M. Mall, A. Wissner, R. Schreiber, J. Kühr, H. H. Seydewitz, M. Brandis, R. Greger and K. Kunzelmann, Role of $K_V LQT1$ in cAMP mediated Cl⁻ secretion in human airways, *Am. J. Respir. Cell Mol. Biol.* **23**, 283-289 (2000).

21. M. Mall, M. Bleich, R. Greger, M. Schürlein, J. Kühr, H. H. Seydewitz, M. Brandis and K. Kunzelmann, Cholinergic ion secretion in human colon requires co-activation by camp, *Am. J. Physiol.* **275**, G1274-G1281 (1998).

22. M. Bleich, N. Riedemann, R. Warth, D. Kerstan, J. Leipziger, M. Hor, W. V. Driessche and R. Greger, Ca^{2+} regulated K⁺ and non-selective cation channels in the basolateral membrane of rat colonic crypt base cells, *Pflugers Arch.* **432**, 1011-1022 (1996).

23. D. Ecke, M. Bleich and R. Greger, Crypt base cells show forskolin-induced Cl⁻ secretion but no cation inward conductance, *Pflugers Arch.* **431**, 427-434 (1996).

24. R. Warth and M. Bleich, K⁺ channels and colonic function, *Rev. Physiol. Biochem. Pharmacol.* **140**, 1-62 (2000).

25. R. Warth, N. Riedemann, M. Bleich, W. Van Driessche, A. E. Busch and R. Greger, The cAMP-regulated and 293B-inhibited K⁺ conductance of rat colonic crypt base cells, *Pflugers Arch.* **432**, 81-88 (1996).

26. D. C. Dawson, Ion channels and colonic salt transport, *Ann. Rev. Physiol.* **53**, 321-339 (1991).

27. W. J. Germann, M. E. Lowy, S. A. Ernst and D. C. Dawson, Differentiation of two distinct K conductances in the basolateral membrane of turtle colon, *J. Gen. Physiol.* **88**, 237-251 (1986).

28. E. Lohrmann, I. Burhoff, R. B. Nitschke, H.-J. Lang, D. Mania, H. C. Englert, M. Hropot, R. Warth, M. Rohm, M. Bleich and R. Greger, A new class of inhibitors of cAMP-mediated Cl⁻ secretion in rabbit colon, acting by the reduction of cAMP-activated K⁺ conductance, *Pflugers Arch.* **429**, 517-530 (1995).

29. F. Grahammer, R. Warth, J. Barhanin, M. Bleich, and M. J. Hug, The small conductance K$^+$ channel KCNQ: expression, function and subunit composition in murine trachea, *J. Biol. Chem.* **276**, 42268-42275 (2001).

30. B. C. Schroeder, S. Waldegger, S. Fehr, M. Bleich, R. Warth, R. Greger, and T. J. Jentsch, A constitutional open potassium channel formed by KCNQ1 and KCNE3, *Nature* **403**, 196-199 (2000).

31. G. Loussouarn, F. Charpentier, R. Mohammad-Panah, K. Kunzelmann, I. Baro, and D. Escande, K$_v$LQT1 potassium channel but not IsK is the molecular target for trans-6-cyano-4-(N-ethylsulfonyl-N-methylamino)-3-hydroxy-2,2-dimethyl-chromane, *Mol. Pharmacol.* **52**, 1131-1136 (1997).

32. G. Romey, B. Attali, C. Chouabe, I. Abitbol, E. Guillemare, J. Barhanin, and M. Lazdunski, Molecular mechanism and functional significance of the MinK control of the KvLQT1 channel activity, *J. Biol. Chem.* **272**, 16713-16716 (1997).

33. M. S. Nielsen, R. Warth, M. Bleich, B. Weyand, and R. Greger, The basolateral Ca^{2+}-dependent K$^+$ channel in rat colonic crypt cells, *Pflugers Arch.* **435**, 267-272 (1998).

34. D. C. Devor and R. A. Frizzell, Modulation of K$^+$ channels by arachidonic acid in T84 cells. I. Inhibition of the Ca^{2+}-dependent K$^+$ channel, *Am. J. Physiol.* **274**, C138-C148 (1998).

35. W. J. Joiner, L. Y. Wang, M. D. Tang, and L. K. Kaczmarek, hSK4, a member of a novel subfamily of calcium-activated potassium channels, *Proc. Natl. Acad. Sci. U.S.A.* **94**, 11013-11018 (1997).

36. T. M. Ishii, C. Silvia, B. Hirschberg, C. T. Bond, J. P. Adelman, and J. Maylie, A human intermediate conductance calcium-activated potassium channel, *Proc. Natl. Acad. Sci. U.S.A.* **94**, 11651-11656 (1997).

37. N. J. Logsdon, J. Kang, J. A. Togo, E. P. Christian, and J. Aiyar, A novel gene, hKCa4, encodes the calcium-activated potassium channel in human T lymphocytes, *J. Biol. Chem.* **272**, 32723-32726 (1997).

38. S. Ghanshani, M. Coleman, P. Gustavsson, A. C. Wu, J. J. Gargus, G. A. Gutman, N. Dahl, H. Mohrenweiser and K. G. Chandy, Human calcium-activated potassium channel gene KCNN4 maps to chromosome 19q13.2 in the region deleted in diamond-blackfan anemia, *Genomics* **51**, 160-161 (1998).

39. A. W. Cuthbert, M. E. Hickman, P. Thorn, and L. J. MacVinish, Activation of Ca^{2+}- and cAMP-sensitive K$^+$ channels in murine colonic epithelia by 1-ethyl-2-benzimidazolone, *Am. J. Physiol.* **277**, C111-C120 (1999).

40. D. C. Devor, A. K. Singh, R. A. Frizzell, and R. J. Bridges, Modulation of Cl$^-$ secretion by benzimidazolones. I. Direct activation of a Ca^{2+}- dependent K$^+$ channel, *Am. J. Physiol.* **271**, L775-L784 (1996).

41. D. C. Devor, A. K. Singh, A. C. Gerlach, R. A. Frizzell and R. J. Bridges, Inhibition of intestinal Cl$^-$ secretion by clotrimazole: direct effect on basolateral membrane K$^+$ channels, *Am. J. Physiol.* **273**, C531-C540 (1997).

42. P. A. Rufo, D. Merlin, M. Riegler, M. H. Ferguson-Maltzman, B. L. Dickinson, C. Brugnara, S. L. Alper, and W. I. Lencer, The antifungal antibiotic, clotrimazole, inhibits chloride secretion by human intestinal T$_{84}$ cells via blockade of distinct basolateral K$^+$ conductances. Demonstration of efficacy in intact rabbit colon and *in vivo* mouse model of cholera, *J. Clin. Invest.* **100**, 3111-3120 (1997).

43. M. J. Stutts, C. M. Canessa, J. C. Olsen, M. Hamrick, J. A. Cohn, B. C. Rossier, and R. C. Boucher, CFTR as a cAMP-dependent regulator of sodium channels, *Science* **269**, 847-850 (1995).

44. M. Mall, A. Hipper, R. Greger and K. Kunzelmann, Wild type but not deltaF508 CFTR inhibits Na$^+$ conductance when coexpressed in *Xenopus* oocytes, *FEBS Letters* **381**, 47-52 (1996).
45. M. Mall, M. Bleich, J. Kühr, M. Brandis, R. Greger and K. Kunzelmann, CFTR - mediated inhibition of amiloride sensitive sodium conductance by CFTR in human colon is defective in cystic fibrosis, *Am. J. Physiol.* **277**, G709-G716 (1999).
46. K. Kunzelmann and M.Mall, Electrolyte transport in the colon: Mechanisms and implications for disease, *Physiol. Rev.* **82**, 245-289 (2002).
47. D. Ecke, M. Bleich, and R. Greger, The amiloride inhibitable Na$^+$ conductance of rat colonic crypt cells is suppressed by forskolin, *Pflugers Arch.* **431**, 984-986 (1996).
48. I. I. Ismailov, M. S. Awayda, B. Jovov, B. K. Berdiev, C. M. Fuller, J. R. Dedman, M. A. Kaetzel, and D. J. Benos, Regulation of epithelial sodium channels by the cystic fibrosis transmembrane conductance regulator, *J. Biol. Chem.* **271**, 4725-4732 (1996).
49. P. M. Quinton, Cystic fibrosis: a disease in electrolyte transport, *FASEB J.* **4**, 2709-2717 (1990).
50. K. Kunzelmann, G. Kiser, R. Schreiber, and J. R. Riordan, Inhibition of epithelial sodium currents by intracellular domains of the cystic fibrosis transmembrane conductance regulator, *FEBS Letters* **400**, 341-344 (1997).
51. A. Boucherot, R. Schreiber, and K. Kunzelmann, Role of CFTR's PDZ- binding domain, NBF1 and Cl$^-$ conductance in inhibition of epithelial Na$^+$ channels in *Xenopus* oocytes, *Biochim. Biophys. Acta* **1515**, 64-71 (2001).
52. J. König, R. Schreiber, T. Voelcker, M. Mall, and K. Kunzelmann, CFTR inhibits ENaC through an increase in the intracellular Cl$^-$ concentration, *EMBO Reports* **2**, 1-5, (2001).
53. K. Kunzelmann and A. Boucherot. Mechanism of the inhibition of epithelial Na$^+$ channels by CFTR and purinergic stimulation, *Kidney International* **60**, 455-461 (2001).
54. A. Hopf, R. Schreiber, R. Greger and K. Kunzelmann, CFTR inhibits the activity of epithelial Na$^+$ channels carrying Liddle's syndrome mutations, *J. Biol. Chem.* **274**, 13894-13899 (1999).
55. M. Briel, R. Greger, and K. Kunzelmann, Cl$^-$ transport by CFTR contributes to the inhibition of epithelial Na$^+$ channels in *Xenopus* ooyctes coexpressing CFTR and ENaC, *J. Physiol. (Lond)* **508.3**, 825-836 (1998).
56. A. Dinudom, J. A. Young and D. I. Cook, Na$^+$ and Cl$^-$ conductances are controlled by cytosolic Cl$^-$ concentration in the intralobular duct cells of mouse mandibular glands, *J. Membrane Biol.* **135**, 289-295 (1993).
57. A. Dinudom, P. Komwatana, J. A. Young, and D. I. Cook, Control of the amiloride-sensitive Na$^+$ current in mouse salivary ducts by intracellular anions is mediated by a G protein, *J. Physiol. (Lond)* **487**, 549-555 (1995).
58. C. Grygorczyk, H. Chabot, D. H. Malinowska, and J. Cuppoletti, Downregulation of ENaC by ClC-2 chloride channel in Xenopus oocytes, *Ped. Pulmonol. Supp.* **22**, Page (2001).
59. K. Kunzelmann, ENaC is inhibited by an increase in the intracellular Cl$^-$ concentration mediated through activation of Cl$^-$ channels, *Pflugers Arch.* **445**, 505-512 (2003).
60. H. P. Ma, S. Saxena and D. G. Warnock, Anionic phospholipids regulate native and expressed ENaC, *J. Biol. Chem.* **277**, 7641-7644 (2002).
61. G. Yue, B. Malik and D. C. Eaton, Phosphatidylinositol 4,5-bisphosphate (PIP$_2$) stimulates epithelial sodium channel activity in A6 cells, *J. Biol. Chem.* **277**, 11965-11969 (2002).

62. N. J. Willumsen and E. H. Larsen, Membrane potentials and intracellular Cl⁻ activity of toad skin epithelium in relation to activation and deactivation of the transepithelial Cl⁻ conductance, *J. Membr. Biol* **94**, 173-190 (1986).

63. N. J. Willumsen, C. W. Davis and R. C. Boucher, Intracellular Cl⁻ activity and cellular Cl⁻ pathways in cultured human airway epithelium, *Am. J. Physiol.* **256**, C1033-C1044 (1989).

64. N. J. Willumsen, C. W. Davis and R. C. Boucher, Cellular Cl⁻ transport in cultured cystic fibrosis airway epithelium, *Am. J. Physiol.* **256**, C1045-C1053 (1989).

65. N. J. Willumsen and R. C. Boucher, Transcellular sodium transport in cultured cystic fibrosis human nasal epithelium, *Am. J. Physiol.* **261**, C332-C341 (1991).

66. M. J. Stutts, C. U. Cotton, J. R. Yankaskas, E. Cheng, M. R. Knowles, J. T. Gatzy and R. C. Boucher, Chloride uptake into cultured airway epithelial cells from cystic fibrosis patients and normal individuals, *Proc. Natl. Acad. Sci. U.S.A.* **82**, 6677-6681 (1985).

67. L. J. Galietta, P. M. Haggie and A. S. Verkman. Green fluorescent protein-based halide indicators with improved chloride and iodide affinities, *FEBS Lett.* **499**, 220-224 (2001).

68. L. J. Galietta, M. F. Springsteel, M. Eda, E. J. Niedzinski, K. By, M. J. Haddadin, M. J. Kurth, M. H. Nantz and A. S. Verkman, Novel CFTR chloride channel activators identified by screening of combinatorial libraries based on flavone and benzoquinolizinium lead compounds, *J. Biol. Chem.* **276**, 19723-19728 (2001).

69. S. Jayaraman, P. Haggie, R. M. Wachter, S. J. Remington and A. S. Verkman, Mechanism and cellular applications of a green fluorescent protein-based halide sensor, *J. Biol. Chem.* **275**, 6047-6050 (2000).

70. M. R. Knowles, L. L. Clarke and R. C. Boucher, Activation by extracellular nucleotides of chloride secretion in the airway epithelia of patients with cystic fibrosis, *N. Engl. J. Med.* **325**, 533-538 (1991).

71. L. L. Clarke and R. C. Boucher, Chloride secretory response to extracellular ATP in human normal and cystic fibrosis nasal epithelia, *Am. J. Physiol.* **263**, C348-C356 (1992).

72. L. L. Clarke, T. C. Chinet and R. C. Boucher, Extracellular ATP stimulates K⁺ secretion across cultured human airway epithelium, *Am. J. Physiol.* **272**, L1084-L1091 (1997).

73. M. J. Stutts, J. G. Fitz, A. M. Paradiso and R. C. Boucher, Multiple modes of regulation of airway epithelial chloride secretion by ATP, *Am. J. Physiol.* **267**, C1442-C1451 (1994).

74. H. A. Brown, E. R. Lazarowski, R. C. Boucher and T. K. Harden, Evidence that UTP and ATP regulate phospholipase C through a common extracellular 5'-nucleotide receptor in human airway epithelial cells, *Mol. Pharmacol.* **40**, 648-655 (1991).

75. I. Butterfield, G. Warhurst, M. N. Jones and G. I. Sandle, Characterization of apical potassium channels induced in rat distal colon during potassium adaptation, *J. Physiol. (Lond).* **501**, 537-547 (1997).

76. O. Zegarra-Moran, O. Sacco, L. Romano, G. A. Rossi and L. J. Galietta, Cl⁻ currents activated by extracellular nucleotides in human bronchial cells, *J. Membr. Biol.* **156**, 297-305 (1997).

77. M. Mall, A. Wissner, J. Kühr, T. Gonska, M. Brandis and K. Kunzelmann, Inhibition of amiloride sensitive epithelial Na⁺ absorption by extracellular nucleotides in human normal and CF airways, *Am. J. Respir. Cell Mol. Biol.* **23**, 755-761 (2000).

78. K. Kunzelmann, R. Schreiber and D. I. Cook, Mechanisms for inhibition of amiloride-sensitive Na⁺ absorption by extracellular nuceotides in mouse trachea, *Pflugers Arch.* **444**, 220-226 (2002).

79. D. Communi, P. Paindavoine, G. A. Place, M. Parmentier and J. M. Boeynaems, Expression of P2Y receptors in cell lines derived from the human lung, *Br. J. Pharmacol.* **127**, 562-568 (1999).

80. E. R. Lazarowski and R. C. Boucher, UTP as an extracellular signaling molecule, *News Physiol. Sci.* **16**, 1-5 (2001).
81. G. R. Dubyak and C. El-Moatassim, Signal transduction via P2-purinergic receptors for extracellular ATP and other nucleotides, *Am. J. Physiol.* **265**, C577-C606 (1993).
82. T. H. Hwang, E. M. Schwiebert and W. B. Guggino, Apical and basolateral ATP stimulates tracheal epithelial chloride secretion via multiple purinergic receptors, *Am. J. Physiol.* **270**, C1611-C1623 (1996).
83. E. R. Lazarowski, A. M. Paradiso, W. C. Watt, T. K. Harden and R. C. Boucher, UDP activates a mucosal-restricted receptor on human nasal epithelial cells that is distinct from the P2Y2 receptor, *Proc. Natl. Acad. Sci. U.S.A.* **94**, 2599-2603 (1997).
84. E. R. Lazarowski, L. Homolya, R. C. Boucher and T. K. Harden, Direct demonstration of mechanically induced release of cellular UTP and its implication for uridine nucleotide receptor activation, *J. Biol. Chem.* **272**, 24348-24354 (1997).
85. L. Homolya, T. H. Steinberg and R. C. Boucher. Cell to Cell Communication in Response to Mechanical Stress via Bilateral Release of ATP and UTP in Polarized Epithelia, *J. Cell. Biol.* **150**, 1349-1360 (2000).
86. W. C. Watt, E. R. Lazarowski and R. C. Boucher, Cystic fibrosis transmembrane regulator independent release of ATP. Its implications for the regulation of P2$^Y_2$ receptors in airway epithelia, *J. Biol. Chem.* **273**, 14053-14058 (1998).
87. M. J. Welsh, Effect of phorbol ester and calcium ionophore on chloride secretion in canine tracheal epithelium, *Am. J. Physiol.* **253**, C828-C834 (1987).
88. M. P. Anderson and M. J. Welsh, Calcium and cAMP activate different chloride channels in the apical membrane of normal and cystic fibrosis epithelia, *Proc. Natl. Acad. Sci. U.S.A.* **88**, 6003-6007 (1991).
89. K. Kunzelmann, S. Kathöfer and R. Greger. Na$^+$ and Cl$^-$ conductances in airway epithelial cells, Increased Na$^+$ conductance in cystic fibrosis, *Pflugers Arch.* **431**, 1-9 (1995).
90. M. Agnel, T. Vermat and J. M. Culouscou, Identification of three novel members of the calcium-dependent chloride channel (CaCC) family predominantly expressed in the digestive tract and trachea, *FEBS Lett.* **455**, 295-301 (1999).
91. A. D. Gruber, K. D. Schreur, H. L. Ji, C. M. Fuller and B. U. Pauli, Molecular cloning and transmembrane structure of hCLCA2 from human lung, trachea, and mammary gland, *Am. J. Physiol.* **276**, C1261-C1270 (1999).
92. Z. Qu, R. W. Wei, W. Mann and H. C. Hartzell, Two bestrophins cloned from Xenopus laevis Oocytes express Ca-activated Cl currents, *J. Biol. Chem* . **278**, 49563-49572 (2003).
93. H. C. Hartzell and Z. Qu, Chloride currents in acutely isolated Xenopus retinal pigment epithelial cells, *J. Physiol.* **549**, 453-469 (2003).
94. T. Koslowsky, T. Hug, D. Ecke, P. Klein, R. Greger, D. C. Gruenert and K. Kunzelmann, Ca^{2+} and swelling induced activation of ion conductances in bronchial epithelial cells, *Pflugers Arch.* **428**, 597-603 (1994).
95. D. C. Devor and J. M. Pilewski, UTP inhibits Na$^+$ absorption in wild-type and DeltaF508 CFTR-expressing human bronchial epithelia, *Am. J. Physiol.* **276**, C827-C837 (1999).
96. J. Thomas, P. Deetjen, W. H. Ko, C. Jacobi and J. Leipziger, P2y$_2$ receptor-mediated inhibition of amiloride-sensitive short circuit current in m-1 mouse cortical collecting duct cells, *J. Membr. Biol.* **183**, 115-124 (2001).
97. H. Lehrmann, J. Thomas, S. J. Kim, C. Jacobi and J. Leipziger, Luminal P2Y2 receptor-mediated inhibition of Na$^+$ absorption in isolated perfused mouse CCD, *J. Am. Soc. Nephrol.* **13**, 10-18 (2002).

98. S. K. Inglis, A. Collett, H. L. McAlroy, S. M. Wilson and R. E. Olver, Effect of luminal nucleotides on Cl⁻ secretion and Na⁺ absorption in distal bronchi, *Pflugers Arch.* **438**, 621-627 (1999).

99. S. J. Ramminger, A. Collett, D. L. Baines, H. Murphie, H. L. McAlroy, R. E. Olver, S. K. Inglis and S. M. Wilson. P2Y₂ receptor-mediated inhibition of ion transport in distal lung epithelial cells, *Br. J. Pharmacol.* **128**, 293-300 (1999).

100. N. Iwase, T. Sasaki, S. Shimura, M. Yamamoto, S. Suzuki and K. Shirato, ATP-induced Cl⁻ secretion with suppressed Na⁺ absorption in rabbit tracheal epithelium, *Respir. Physiol.* **107**, 173-180 (1997).

101. H. P. Ma, L. Li, Z. H. Zhou, D. C. Eaton and D. G. Warnock, ATP masks stretch activation of epithelial sodium channels in A6 distal nephron cells, *Am. J. Physiol.* **282**, F501-F505 (2002).

102. D. W. Hilgemann, S. Feng and C. Nasuhoglu, The complex and intriguing lives of PIP2 with ion channels and transporters, *Sci. STKE* **2001**, RE19 (2001).

103. K. Kunzelmann and M. Mall, Pharmacotherapy of the Ion Transport Defect in Cystic Fibrosis, Potential Role of P2Y2 Receptor Agonists, *Am. J. Resp. Med.* **2**, 299-399 (2003).

104. B. Heinke, R. Ribeiro and M. Diener, Involvement of calmodulin and protein kinase C in the regulation of K⁺ transport by carbachol across the rat distal colon, *Eur. J. Pharmacol.* **377**, 75-80 (1999).

105. A. K. Singh, D. C. Devor, A. C. Gerlach, M. Gondor, J. M. Pilewski and R. J. Bridges, Stimulation of Cl⁻ secretion by chlorzoxazone, *J. Pharmacol. Exp. Ther.* **292**, 778-787 (2000).

106. H. Garty and L. G. Palmer, Epithelial sodium channels, Function, structure and regulation, *Physiol. Rev.* **77**, 359-396 (1997).

107. M.R. Knowles, K. N. Olivier, K. W. Hohneker, J. Robinson, W. D. Bennett and R. C. Boucher, Pharmacologic treatment of abnormal ion transport in the airway epithelium in cystic fibrosis, *Chest* **107**, 71S-76S (1995).

108. R. P. Tomkiewicz, E. M. App, J. G. Zayas, O. Ramirez, N. Church, R. C. Boucher, M. R. Knowles and M. King, Amiloride inhalation therapy in cystic fibrosis. Influence on ion content, hydration, and rheology of sputum, *Am. Rev. Respir. Dis.* **148**, 1002-1007 (1993).

109. M. R. Knowles, N. L. Church, W. E. Waltner, J. R. Yankaskas, P. Gilligan, M. King, L. J. Edwards, R. W. Helms and R. C. Boucher, A pilot study of aerosolized amiloride for the treatment of lung disease in cystic fibrosis, *N. Engl. J. Med.* **322**, 1189-1194 (1990).

110. A. Graham, A. Hasani, E. W. Alton, G. P. Martin, C. Marriott, M. E. Hodson, S. W. Clarke and D. M. Geddes, No added benefit from nebulized amiloride in patients with cystic fibrosis, *Eur. Respir. J.* **6**, 1243-1248 (1993).

111. S. Ghosal, C. J. Taylor, W. H. Colledge, R. Ratcliff and M. J. Evans, Sodium channel blockers and uridine triphosphate, effects on nasal potential difference in cystic fibrosis mice, *Eur. Respir. J.* **15**, 146-150 (2000).

112. W. Pendergast, B. R. Yerxa, J. G. Douglass, S. R. Shaver, R. W. Dougherty, C. C. Redick, I. F. Sims and J. L. Rideout, Synthesis and P2Y receptor activity of a series of uridine dinucleoside 5'-polyphosphates, *Bioorg. Med. Chem. Lett.* **11**, 157-160 (2001).

113. J. R. Sabater, Y. M. Mao, C. Shaffer, M. K. James, T. G. O'Riordan and W. M. Abraham, Aerosolization of P2Y₂-receptor agonists enhances mucociliary clearance in sheep, *J. Appl. Physiol.* **87**, 2191-2196 (1999).

114. S. D. Guile, F. Ince, A. H. Ingall, N. D. Kindon, P. Meghani and M. P. Mortimore, The medicinal chemistry of the P2 receptor family, *Prog. Med. Chem.* **38**, 115-187 (2001).

115. D. Mathews, D. Kellerman, J. Gorden, C. Johnson and R. Evans, INS37217, a novel P2Y2 receptor agonist, being developed for the treatment of cystic fibrosis, results from

initial phase 1 study in normal volunteers, *European Cystic Fibrosis Conference 2001 June 6-9; Vienna, Austria* (2002).

116. P. G. Noone, N. Hamblett, F. Accurso, M. L. Aitken, M. Boyle, M. Dovey, R. Gibson, C. Johnson, D. Kellerman, M. W. Konstan, L. Milgram, J. Mundahl, G. Retsch-Bogort, D. Rodman, J. Williams-Warren, R. W. Wilmott, P. Zeitlin and B. Ramsey, Safety of aerosolized INS 365 in patients with mild to moderate cystic fibrosis, results of a phase I multi-center study, *Pediatr. Pulmonol.* **32**, 122-128 (2001).

Chapter 3

ION CHANNELS IN THE APICAL MEMBRANE: ROLE OF ELECTRICAL COUPLING ON TRANSEPITHELIAL TRANSPORT

Jean-Daniel Horisberger
Institut de Pharmacologie et de Toxicologie, Université Lausanne, Bugnon 27, CH-1005 Lausanne, Switzerland. Tel.: +41 21 692 5362; Fax +41 21 692 5355; e-mail Jean-Daniel.Horisberger@ipharm.unil.ch

1. INTRODUCTION

The role of many epithelia is to secrete or absorb fluid, and this function is usually carried out by active transport of NaCl followed by passive osmotic water flow. In addition to ion pumps and coupled transport system, several types of channel (Na^+, K^+, Cl^- channels) are responsible for the transepithelial ion transport and these channels may be present in parallel in the apical membrane of epithelial cells. Because the channels carry an ionic current, each of them modifies the voltage of the apical membrane and influences the driving force for ion flow through the other channels present in the same membrane. In addition, when the epithelium is maintained under open circuit conditions, each conductive or rheogenic element also influences the potential across the whole epithelium and across the controlateral membrane because of the current loop flowing through the cells and the tight junctions.[1] Because of the reciprocal influence of channels and other electrogenic transporters it is not always easy to predict the direction and the magnitude of ion flow in a system that includes several channels, pumps and transporters.

The aim of the present study was to explore the interaction of Na^+, Cl^- and K^+ conductances that may be present and active in the apical membrane of a NaCl transporting epithelium, and evaluate the consequences of these interactions on transepithelial ion fluxes in a quantitative manner. The specific purpose of these simulations was to better understand the interactions of the epithelial sodium channel, ENaC, with the chloride conductance that is provided by the activated CFTR in airways or renal epithelia, but the model can apply to many other epithelia. It has to be noted that the results of this type of model apply only under the conditions that these conductances are present in the apical membrane of the same cell, or possibly in the apical membrane of adjacent but electrically highly coupled cells. This model would not apply to tissues in which ENaC and CFTR are expressed largely in different cells, such as it is the case for the colon epithelium, where ENaC is mostly expressed in surface cells, while CFTR is rather abundant at the bottom of the crypts.[2-4]

2.   METHODS

The model used for the simulations will be only briefly described here, as it has been presented in details earlier[5] and has undergone only a few minor modifications for the present work. The elements of the epithelial cell model are illustrated in the scheme of Figure 1a and include Na^+, K^+ and Cl^- conductances in the apical membrane, and in the basolateral membrane K^+ and Cl^- conductances, a Na,K pump with a fixed 3 Na^+ for 2 K^+ stoichiometry and a $Na^+/K^+/2Cl^-$ cotransport system. The paracellular shunt pathway provides passive permeability for Na^+, K^+ and Cl^- ions.

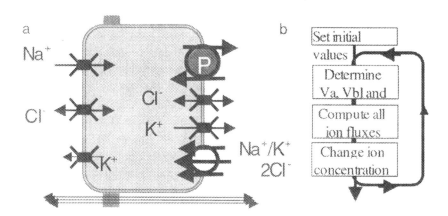

Figure 1. a) Scheme showing all the functional elements of the epithelial cell model, namely the ionic conductances, the Na,K pump (P) and the $Na^+/K^+/2Cl^-$ cotransport system. The paracellular pathway includes Na^+, K^+ and Cl^- conductances. b) Flow chart illustrating the sequence of calculations in the model program.

The variables of the model are the apical (Va) and basolateral (Vbl) membrane potentials, the transepithelial potential (Vte = Va + Vbl), and the ion concentrations in the intracellular and apical compartment (in these calculations the basolateral compartment was assumed to have an infinite volume and thus have stable ion concentrations). The parameters of the model, namely the ionic permeability for each conductance, the transport parameters for the Na,K pump and the $Na^+/K^+/2Cl^-$ cotransporter, are described in Table 1 with the baseline values that were attributed to these parameters.

The principle of the calculation is illustrated in the flowchart of Figure 1b. After setting initial values for each variable, a sequence of three steps is repeated for a short time interval (typically 1 s) i) the membrane and transepithelial potentials are first calculated using a numerical solution search for the membrane potentials allowing for electroneutrality, ii) the ion fluxes through each transport system across the apical and basolateral membrane and across the paracellular pathway are calculated taking into account the ion concentrations and the membrane or transepithelial potential, iii) new values of the ion concentrations of the apical fluid and intracellular

Table 1. Baseline parameters used in two set of simulations.

Parameters		"absorptive" epithelium	"secretory" epithelium		Units
apical membrane conductances [a]	pNa_a	0.8	0.1	10^{-6}	cm/s
	pK_a	0.01	0.01	10^{-6}	cm/s
	pCl_a	0.5	2	10^{-6}	cm/s
basolateral membrane conductances [a]	pK_{bl}	4	4	10^{-6}	cm/s
	pCl_{bl}	1	1	10^{-6}	cm/s
Na,K pump parameters [b]	iP_{max}	20	20		$\mu A/cm^2$
	kNa_i	10	10		mM
	nHill	3	3		nHill
Na/K/2Cl cotransporter [c]	trCl	60	60		pmol/ s.cm^2
paracellular shunt conductances [a]	pNa_s	0.01	3	10^{-6}	cm/s
	pCl_s	0.4	0.4	10^{-6}	cm/s
	pK_s	0.1	0.1	10^{-6}	cm/s

[a] the magnitude of the ion conductances are expressed permeabilities
[b] the Na,K-pump parameters are the maximal activity expressed as the maximal Na,K-pump current iP_{max} (one unitary charge for a 3 Na^+ to 2 K^+ exchange), the apparent affinity for intracellular Na^+ and a Hill coefficient.
[c] the Na/K/2Cl cotransporter was assumed to function at a constant rate independently of the ion concentrations.

compartment are calculated from the ion fluxes and the volume of the compartment. The volumes of the apical and intracellular compartments are set to be constant, meaning that there are no water movements. All the calculations were performed using the Mathematica® software (Wolfram Research, Champain, IL, USA). The extracellular concentrations were set to Na^+ 130 mM, K^+ 4 mM, and Cl^- 134 mM.

All membrane conductances were assumed to conform to the Goldman-Hodgkin-Katz flux equation, except for the basolateral membrane conductance for which an inward rectifying factor has been added, according to the experimental evidence that this conductance is rather inward rectifying.[6] A difference from the model published earlier[5] is the fact that the paracellular Na, K^+ and Cl^- fluxes were also computed from the Goldman-Hodgkin-Katz equation.

Two versions of the program allow simulating *current clamp conditions*, in which the transepithelial current was set to 0 except for 1-s current injection used to compute the membrane and transepithelial conductances, or *voltage clamp conditions*, in which the transepithelial potential was set to 0, except for 1-s voltage perturbation used to compute the membrane conductances.

3.   RESULTS AND DISCUSSION

Three main types of experimental conditions were examined. First conditions simulating the standard Ussing chamber type of experiments in which the relatively large volumes of the apical and basolateral compartment preclude any significant changes in the ionic composition of both of these compartments and this situation was studied either under voltage clamp or under current clamp conditions. These simulations were allowed to proceed until a steady state was reached, namely that stable membrane potentials and intracellular ionic concentrations were reached. The electrophysiological characteristics (membrane and transepithelial potentials, intracellular ion concentrations, membrane and transepithelial resistances) at steady state under open circuit conditions are shown in Table 2. Another condition was studied that represents the experimental conditions in which the apical compartment has a small volume (10 $\mu l/cm^2$) and transepithelial fluxes result in significant changes in the ionic concentration of the apical compartment. These simulations were also allowed to proceed until a steady state was reached, in which stable membrane potentials and intracellular and apical compartment ionic concentrations were reached, i.e. until there was no transepithelial net ion fluxes anymore (even though finite transcellular and paracellular fluxes of similar magnitude but opposite direction might still be present).

Table 2. Electrophysiological characteristics of the epithelia modeled according to the parameters shown in Table 1.

Variables		"absorptive" epithelium	"secretory" epithelium	units
transepithelial and membrane potentials	Vte	-49	-6.1	mV
	Va	17	57	mV
	Vbl	-67	-63	mV
intracellular ion concentrations	Na_i	6.6	5.6	mM
	K_i	105	112	mM
	Cl_i	21.7	28.3	mM
transepithelial and membrane resistances	Rte	2292	520	Ω/cm^2
	Ra	2711	2767	Ω/cm^2
	Rbl	1293	1619	Ω/cm^2
	Rsh	4777	593	Ω/cm^2

3.1 Role of the apical Na^+ and Cl^- conductances in transepithelial NaCl fluxes in an absorptive type of epithelial cell

I first examined the effect of changing the apical membrane conductances on the transport properties of an absorptive type of epithelium, starting with modification of the Na^+ conductance to test the model. The parameters chosen to represent an absorptive epithelium are shown in the first column in Table 1. As expected, increasing the apical membrane Na^+ conductance increase the transepithelial potential while partially depolarizing the basolateral membrane (Figure 1, left panel). Under voltage clamp conditions, there was a large increase of the short circuit current that however saturated when the apical membrane conductance reached about 2 $mS.cm^{-2}$. When the apical compartment concentrations were allowed to equilibrate until no net transport occurred, the capacity to create a large transepithelial Na^+ gradient (a low Na^+ concentration in the apical compartment) was strongly related to the magnitude of the Na^+ conductance (Figure 1, right panel).

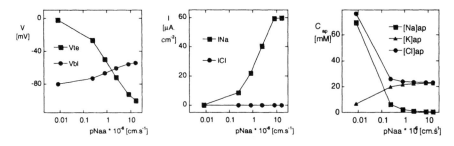

Figure 2. Effects of apical membrane Na^+ permeability (PNaa) on transepithelial and basolateral membrane potentials (Vte, Vbl, current clamp conditions), Na^+ and Cl^- transcellular current (INa, ICl, voltage clamp conditions) and limiting transepithelial Na^+, K^+, and Cl^- gradients: apical compartment Na^+, K^+, and Cl^- concentrations (Na_ap, K_ap, Cl_ap, current clamp conditions, limited apical volume). Potential, current and concentration values are reported as a function of PNaa. All other parameters are kept constant with the values indicated in Table 1, "absorptive epithelium" column.

Increasing the Cl^- conductance of the apical membrane (pCl_a) had more interesting effects. Although the magnitude of pCl_a did not influence the short circuit current measured under voltage clamp conditions (data not shown), a large pCl_a depolarized the transepithelial potential while hyperpolarizing the basolateral membrane (Figure 3, upper panel). Under transepithelial current clamp, increasing pCl_a resulted in larger Na^+ and Cl^- absortive fluxes (Figure 3, lower panel). The limiting transepithelial gradient was not sensitive to the size of the apical membrane Cl^- conductance (data not shown).

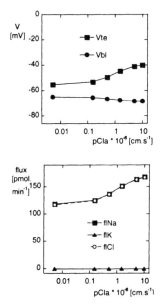

Figure 3. Effects of apical membrane Cl^- permeability (PCla) on transepithelial and basolateral membrane potentials (Vte, Vbl) and on transepithelial Na^+ and Cl^- fluxes under current clamp conditions. Potential or fluxes values (for 1 cm^2) are reported as a function of PCla. All other parameters are kept constant with the values indicated in Table 2, "absorptive" epithelium column.

3.2 Parameters determining the absorptive and secretory function of the epithelium

In a second set of experiments, I examined the effect of several parameters on the transepithelial fluxes with baseline conditions that would allow for net NaCl absorption or secretion. The parameters chosen for these experiments are shown in the second column, entitled "secretory epithelium" of Table 1. Figure 4 (left panel) shows that the activity of the basolateral $Na^+/K^+/2Cl^-$ cotransporter on transepithelial fluxes had a strong influence of the vectorial solute transport that shifted from a reabsortive direction to large secretory fluxes when its activity was elevated while all other parameters were kept constant.

The selectivity of the paracellular shunt conductance was also very important in determining the direction of the net NaCl transport. The effect of modulating the paracellular shunt Na^+ conductance (middle panel) and Cl^- conductance (right panel) are also shown in Figure 4. It is obvious that large sodium permeability is necessary to obtain NaCl secretion while, while increasing chloride permeability can reduce solute secretion and even reverse the flux to a net luminal to serosal transepithelial NaCl transport.

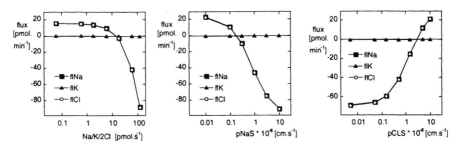

Figure 4. Effect of paracellular Na^+ and Cl^- permeability (pNaS and pClS) and $Na^+/K^+/2Cl^-$ cotransporter activity on the transepithelial Na^+ and Cl^- fluxes under open circuit conditions. Transepithelial fluxes are reported as a function of the Na^+ and Cl^- apical membrane permeability (PNaa, PCla) or of the transport rate through the $Na^+/K^+/2Cl^-$ cotransporter. All other parameters are kept constant with the values indicated in Table 2, "secretory epithelium" column. Positive flux values indicate an absorptive direction while negative values indicate a secretion.

4. CONCLUSIONS

In an "absorptive" type of epithelium we find, not surprisingly, that either the short circuit current or the steady state transepithelial NaCl flux or the limiting transepithelial Na^+ gradient are highly dependent on the apical membrane Na^+ conductance, i.e. on the density of open ENaC in the apical membrane. The values obtained for the limiting transepithelial Na^+ gradient are compatible with those observed under similar conditions, i.e. maximally stimulated Na^+ transport such as those reported for aldosterone treated rats[7] for which the concentration of sodium in urine was found around 1 or 2 mM and some times below 1 mM (unpublished personal observations).

The effect of changing the apical membrane Cl^- permeability may be more interesting. First, the size of the apical membrane Cl^- conductance had practically no effect either on the short circuit current, or on the limiting transepithelial Na^+ gradient. Increasing the apical membrane Cl^- conductance had however a physiologically significant effect on the transepithelial NaCl fluxes measured under current clamp conditions. Activating an apical Cl^- conductance resulted in an *increased* NaCl absorption when the apical NaCl concentration remains high because the luminal fluid flow rate is fast enough to prevent significant concentration changes or because the water permeability is large enough to allow isotonic fluid reabsorption. This observation indicates that the shift from a reabsorptive to a secretory type of function cannot be achieved by only activating CFTR in the apical membrane. The absence of influence of the apical Cl^- conductance on the limiting NaCl gradient and on the steady state short circuit current suggests that the difference between the presence or the absence of an active apical Cl^- conductance might be difficult to demonstrate in an absorptive epithelium and may be evident only under specific conditions, namely low water permeability and high luminal fluid flow rate. Such conditions would be observed for the kidney in animals under sodium restriction and water diuresis. Although there is good evidence for the presence of CFTR in the distal nephron,[8,9] no obvious defect in NaCl urinary excretion has been described in CF patients. It might be interesting to look for a difference of NaCl transport in the kidney between CF animal models and normal animals under specific conditions.

The second series of simulations point the important role of the ionic selectivity of the paracellular shunt pathway for the net direction, reabsorptive or secretory, of the NaCl transepithelial flux as well as the role of the basolateral $Na^+/K^+/2Cl^-$ cotransport that allows to accumulate Cl^- in the cell to a concentration above its equilibrium potential across the apical membrane. Most of the experimental work on the balance between fluid secretion and reabsorption by airway epithelia has focused on the control of ENaC and CFTR. The present results suggest that this balance may depend not only on the control of these two ion channels but also importantly on the conductive properties of the paracellular pathway, for which not so many experimental data are available.

REFERENCES

1. E. L. Boulpaep and H. Sackin, Equivalent electrical circuit analysis and rheogenic pump in epithelia, *Fed. Proc.* **38**, 2030-2036 (1979).
2. C. Duc, N. Farman, C. M. Canessa, J.-P. Bonvalet, and B. C. Rossier, Cell-specific expression of epithelial sodium channel α, β, and gamma subunits in aldosterone-responsive epithelia from the rat: Localization by in situ hybridization and immunocytochemistry, *J. Cell Biol.* **127**, 1907-1921 (1994).
3. D. Ecke, M. Bleich, and R. Greger, The amiloride inhibitable Na^+ conductance of rat colonic crypt cells is suppressed by forskolin, *Pflugers Arch.* **431**(6), 984-986 (1996).
4. A. Kockerling, D. Sorgenfrei, and M. Fromm, Electrogenic Na^+ absorption of rat distal colon is confined to surface epithelium: a voltage-scanning study, *Am. J. Physiol. Cell Physiol.* **264**, C1285-C1293 (1996).
5. J.-D. Horisberger, ENaC-CFTR interactions: the role of electrical coupling explored in an epithelial cell model, *Pflugers Arch.* **445**(4), 522-528 (2003).
6. M.-C. Broillet and J.-D. Horisberger, Basolateral membrane conductance of A6 cells, *J. Membrane Biol.* **124**, 1-12 (1991).
7. J.-D. Horisberger and J. Diezi, Effects of mineralocorticoids on Na^+ and K^+ excretion in the adrenalectomized rat, *Am. J. Physiol.* **245**, F89-F99 (1983).
8. J. P. D. Van Huyen, M. Bens, J. Teulon, and A. Vandewalle, Vasopressin-stimulated chloride transport in transimmortalized mouse cell lines derived from the distal convoluted tubule and cortical and inner medullary collecting ducts, *Neph. Dial. Transplantation* **16**(2), 238-245 (2001).
9. B. Letz and C. Korbmacher, cAMP stimulates CFTR-like Cl^- channels and inhibits amiloride-sensitive Na^+ channels in mouse CCD cells, *Am. J. Physiol. Cell Physiol.* **41**(2), C-C (1997).

Chapter 4

ION CHANNELS IN SECRETORY GRANULES OF THE PANCREAS: MOLECULAR IDENTIFICATION AND THEIR ROLE IN REGULATED SECRETION

Frank Thévenod

Department of Physiology & Pathophysiology, University of Witten/Herdecke, D-58448 Witten, Germany. Tel.: +49 (0) 2302 669-221, Fax: +49 (0) 2302 669-182, E-mail: frank.thevenod@uni-wh.de

1. INTRODUCTION

Exocrine and endocrine cells, such as pancreatic acinar and beta-cells, are morphologically characterized by the presence of intracellular membrane-bound vesicles (or "granules") that secrete their content into the extracellular milieu in a regulated manner. Secretion takes place as a two-step process: 1) exocytosis and 2) discharge of solute molecules and stored macromolecular secretory products - digestive proenzymes (the "zymogens") in pancreatic acinar cells and insulin in pancreatic beta-cells – into the cell exterior.

A prerequisite of this process is a "fusion-fission" reaction between the membrane of secretory granules and the plasma membrane (PM) of secretory cells. Prior to exocytosis, the granules undergo a "docking" reaction at specific release sites, which involves the binding of several granule- and PM-associated complementary proteins (for review, see ref. 1). This is followed by a "priming" reaction, which requires metabolic energy and provides competence of docked granules for membrane fusion and exocytosis. A specific signal, e.g. an increase of intracellular Ca^{2+} concentration ($[Ca^{2+}]_i$), then stimulates exocytosis, which is followed by the release of the granule matrix. This discharge process appears to be triggered by specific signaling molecules, temporally distinct from and not obligatorily coupled to exocytosis.[2,3] Recent biochemical and biophysical studies in pancreatic acinar and insulin-secreting beta-cells provide compelling evidence that ion fluxes through granule ion channels modulate exocytosis and/or the release of macromolecular secretory products.

2.   ION CHANNELS IN SECRETORY GRANULES OF PANCREATIC ACINAR CELLS

Secretion by the exocrine pancreas is carried out by two morphologically and functionally distinct epithelia, the acini and ducts. In acinar cells, an increase   intracellular calcium levels ($[Ca^{2+}]_i$) evoked by the secretagogues acetylcholine (ACh) or cholecystokinin (CCK) leads to the secretion of a near neutral primary fluid by Na^+-coupled secondary active Cl^- transport. Concomitantly digestive enzymes, which are stored as pro-enzymes in zymogen granules (ZG) at the apex of the cells, are released into the lumen. This primary secretion is subsequently modified by downstream duct cells, which generate the HCO_3^--rich pancreatic juice.

It is well established that in addition to Ca^{2+}-sensitive second messenger molecules, several Ca^{2+}-sensitive proteins interact at different stages to promote fusion, exocytosis, and secretion of the ZG contents.[4] Membrane fusion requires the formation of complexes between complementary proteins in the ZG membrane (v-SNAREs) and the target plasma membrane (PM) (t-SNAREs) of acinar cells,[5,6] whose role is to bring granular and target membranes close together. As a consequence of fusion, components of the ZG membrane may be inserted into the PM. Anion channels located at the apical membrane are integral to the secretion of fluid and electrolytes from secretory epithelia. The best characterized of these channels is the cAMP-sensitive cystic fibrosis transmembrane conductance regulator or CFTR (ABCC7) protein. CFTR is expressed in membranes of mucin granules in goblet cells,[7] but in the pancreas it is primarily localized to the ducts.[8] Ca^{2+}-dependent secretion of NaCl is thought to be mediated by Ca^{2+}-sensitive Cl^- channels in the apical PM,[9] but it may also involve insertion of Ca^{2+}-activated anion channels in the membrane of ZG into the apical PM.[10]

Early studies have shown that enzyme secretion evoked by Ca^{2+}-dependent secretagogues in permeabilized pancreatic acini requires the presence of Cl^- and K^+ in the cytosol and is abolished by application of Cl^- and K^+ channel blockers.[11] This led to the hypothesis that ion conductances in ZG membranes (ZGM) play a major role in modulating regulated secretion (for review, see Ref. 12). Subsequently, hormonally regulated anion and cation conductive pathways have been identified in the membrane of isolated ZG using a quantitative *in vitro* assay to measure macroscopic ion fluxes, based on osmotic swelling and end-point measurements of granular lysis.[12] These observations were therefore consistent with the hypothesis that activation of regulated ion conductive pathways in ZG membranes play a significant role in modulating secretion triggered by secretagogues.

As a first step towards the identification of the ion channel proteins associated with these ZG conductive pathways, a pharmacological "footprinting" was carried out. Inhibitors of K^+ and Cl^- channels, such as Ba^{2+} or 4,4'-diisothiocyanatostilbene-2, 2'-disulfonic acid (DIDS), inhibited K^+ and Cl^- conductive pathways, respectively.[12,13] Glyburide (glibenclamide), quinidine, or ATP binding blocked K^+ conductance and increased Cl^- conductance.[12,14] Furthermore, evidence was obtained that the effect of these compounds results from their binding to a 65-kDa multidrug resistance P-glycoprotein (ABCB1; mdr1) gene product, which regulates Cl^- and K^+ conductances.[15,16]

The first evidence for the expression of a cloned Cl^- channel in ZG was provided by Carew and Thorn.[17] They recorded ClC-2-like Cl^- currents in pig pancreatic acinar cells by the whole-cell patch-clamp technique. Immunohistochemical localization with a ClC-2 antibody revealed expression in both, apical PM and ZG. This suggested that the channel remains functional in the plasma membrane after exocytosis and that it may function as a Cl^- efflux pathway in pancreatic acinar cells.

2.1   A CLCA protein may account for Ca^{2+}-activated HCO_3^- conductance in ZG[18]

A CLCA channel family member could be a potential candidate for a ZG anion conductive pathway that is activated by micromolar concentrations of Ca^{2+}. This family now consists of at least ten isoforms from different species, including four human and four murine homologs (for review, see Ref. 19). These putative anion channels are gated by Ca^{2+} and mostly expressed in the PM of epithelial tissues. When heterologously expressed in HEK 293 cells, all isoforms of the CLCA (chloride channel, Ca^{2+}-activated) family investigated so far (hCLCA1, hCLCA2, mCLCA1 and bCLCA1) induced a Ca^{2+}-sensitive anion conductance with an $I^- > Cl^-$ selectivity profile, a linear I-V-relationship and a 25 pS single-channel conductance that can be blocked by 4,4'-diisothiocyanatostilbene-2,2'-disulfonic acid (DIDS) and the reducing agent dithiothreitol (DTT), consistent with the hypothesis that the functional channel protein is a multimer of homomeric subunits (for review, see ref. 19,20). So far there had been no evidence to suggest an intracellular localization of CLCA channels. However, recently Leverkoehne and Gruber have identified mCLCA3 (mgob-5) in the membrane of mucin granules of goblet cells from intestinal, respiratory, and uterine epithelia.[21]

Because *in situ* hybridization studies also demonstrated mCLCA1/2 expression in the acini of the mouse pancreas,[22] we investigated the expression, localization and function of CLCA1 in rat pancreatic acinar cells. Using primers derived from the sequence of mouse CLCA1, we have generated a RT-PCR product with rat pancreatic mRNA, which exhibits 81%, 77%, and 57% amino acid similarity to the three mouse isoforms mCLCA-1, -2, and -3 (mgob-5), respectively.[18] Immunofluorescence light microscopy with an antibody against a 38-kDa subunit of bovine CLCA1 showed labeling of acinar cells in the granular area. This observation was confirmed by pre-embedding electron microscopy immunogold labeling of ZG membranes.[18] The pattern of immunoreactive bands obtained in ZG membranes by SDS-PAGE and immunoblotting suggests that rat pancreatic CLCA also undergoes posttranslational modification to form a heterodimer consisting of a 90-kDa and a 30-40-kDa subunit, as proposed for other members of this CLCA protein family.[19] Surprisingly, functional studies in isolated ZG did not show any activation of the Cl⁻ conductive pathway by low micromolar [Ca^{2+}]. However, when Cl⁻ was replaced by I⁻ or HCO_3^- the conductance was increased by low micromolar [Ca^{2+}]. The [Ca^{2+}] required for activation of the anion conductive pathway with I⁻ or HCO_3^- as permeant anions was in the range of 2.5-50μM, whereas [Ca^{2+}] above 100μM was inhibitory. This is consistent with a similar biphasic effect of Ca^{2+} observed in previous studies with bovine CLCA1 reconstituted into planar lipid bilayers.[20] Inhibitors of the CLCA-channels, H_2-DIDS and DTT, inhibited Ca^{2+}-activated I⁻ and HCO_3^- conductances, whereas in the absence of Ca^{2+} both compounds were without effect.[18] In contrast the Ca^{2+} concentrations required for activation of the ZG anion conductance with Cl⁻ as anion exceeded 100μM. It is interesting to note that the physiological anion that permeates the Ca^{2+}-sensitive anion conductance is not Cl⁻ but HCO_3^-. While current models suggest that luminal CFTR and a Cl⁻/ HCO_3^- exchanger are key players in the process of ductal HCO_3^- secretion, little attention has been drawn to the role of acinar HCO_3^- secretion, particularly in the context of hydration, disaggregation and decondensation of digestive pro-enzymes stored in secretory granules. Moreover, it has been shown that alkalinization of the pancreatic acinar lumen enhances retrieval of exocytotic membranes by cleavage of GPI-anchored proteins.[23] This suggests that changes in luminal HCO_3^- concentration mediated by activation of a ZG HCO_3^--permeable and Ca^{2+}-sensitive anion channel could also affect acinar membrane dynamics by enhancing apical endocytosis (see Figure 1).

Our hypothesis that a CLCA protein may be involved in HCO_3^- transport in ZG to stimulate enzyme secretion by pancreatic acinar cells is particularly attractive in the context of the concept that a Ca^{2+}-activated anion conductance (CaCC) - possibly mediated by CLCA - could represent a "rescue" pathway in cystic fibrosis (CF) and in mouse models of CF with mild pancreatic insufficiency, in which the activity of the CaCC is upregulated under circumstances where cAMP-dependent Cl^- secretion is absent or defective (for review, see ref. 24). Thus future studies need to establish the identity and functional role of CLCA1/2 in acinar cells from normal and CF pancreas.

2.2 Activation of a chromanol-sensitive KCNQ1 K^+ channel in ZG is required for enzyme secretion

Two monovalent cation conductive pathways contribute to K^+ fluxes into ZG: A non-selective monovalent cation conductive pathway is blocked by flufenamic acid,[14] whereas a K^+ selective conductive pathway is blocked by ATP and glibenclamide[13] and therefore appears to have some properties of K_{ATP} channels. In preliminary experiments, we have succeeded to reconstitute ATP-sensitive K^+ channels in ZG membrane vesicles using the planar bilayer technique (F. Thévenod and A. Szewczyk, unpublished results), thus confirming the results obtained with the macroscopic ion flux approach. However, $K_{ir6.2}$, the pore forming subunit of K_{ATP} channels, is not expressed in rat pancreatic acini.[25] KCNQ1 (K_vLQT1) may be a candidate for the ZG K^+ channel (for review, see ref. 26). *In situ* hybridization studies have shown that KCNQ1 and KCNE1 are expressed in rodent pancreatic acini.[27] In some epithelial tissues, KCNQ1 K^+ channels were found to be selectively inhibited by the chromanol 293B, which binds to KCNQ1.[28]

In rat pancreatic acini, 293B (10μM) completely inhibited K^+ conductance, whereas the non-selective and Cl^- conductances were not affected by up to 100μM of the drug. Though 293B is not absolutely specific for KCNQ1, higher concentrations of the drugs are required to inhibit other ion channels.[28] 293B also blocked CCK-OP-stimulated amylase secretion from permeabilized rat pancreatic acini in a concentration dependent manner (EC_{50} about 10μM), whereas basal amylase release was not changed. Using an antibody against the cytosolic N-terminus of KCNQ1, a protein of about 80kDa was detected in ZG membranes and PM of rat pancreas, which is consistent with its predicted M_r based on a protein of 669 amino acids. It remains to be investigated whether KNCQ1 co-assembles with a regulatory subunit distinct from KCNE1, as described for other tissues,[26] to account for the unusual functional properties of ZG K^+ conductance, such as block by ATP or glibenclamide.

The presence of ion channel proteins in the membrane of ZG lends support to the hypothesis that following exocytosis elicited by physiological stimuli ZG ion channels modulate the release of stored digestive enzymes (see Figure 1). This concept is strengthened by studies using atomic force microscopy to study ZG exocytosis in single pancreatic acinar cells and osmotic swelling of isolated ZG.[29,30] These reports proposed that granule swelling induced by activation of ZG ion channels takes place after exocytosis to prevent granule collapse and/or to ensure "kiss-and-run" recycling of secretory granules (Figure 1).[31]

3.   ION CHANNELS IN SECRETORY GRANULES OF PANCREATIC BETA-CELLS

Insulin is produced in the beta-cells of the islet of Langerhans, where it is stored in secretory granules until its release into the bloodstream by regulated exocytosis. Beta-cells are electrically active and use this property to sense elevated blood levels of metabolic fuels and to couple them to insulin release. The transduction pathway linking glucose metabolism to changes of the electrical activity of beta-cells to induce insulin secretion is relatively well understood. Glucose is taken up by the cells via the glucose carrier GLUT-2 and metabolized to ATP in mitochondria. The increase in ATP/ADP ratio leads to closure of ATP-sensitive K^+ channels (K_{ATP}-channels) in the plasma membrane. Closure of K_{ATP}-channels leads to a depolarization of the beta-cell and to activation of voltage-gated L-type Ca^{2+}-channels that further accentuates the depolarization and initiates action potentials. Influx of Ca^{2+} through these channels leads to an increase of the cytoplasmic Ca^{2+} concentration, which then stimulates exocytosis of the insulin-containing granules and the release of insulin.[3,32]

The mechanisms underlying the final steps of exocytosis and insulin release are less well established. Unlike ZG of pancreatic acinar cells, the packaged secretory granules gradually acidify to allow further processing of insulin. The granules are stored throughout the cytosol and eventually translocated to release sites near the PM. The fusion of the granules with the PM is triggered by Ca^{2+} and controlled by Ca^{2+}-dependent and -independent docking and fusion proteins, which include SNARE proteins.[1,33] Kinetic modeling of exocytosis has shown that only a small fraction of the granules of a beta-cell (~1-5%, also referred to as readily releasable pool) (RRP) are in a "primed" state, which makes them immediately available for exocytosis upon Ca^{2+} influx. The remaining granules form a "reserve" pool. This classification into two distinct pools correlates with biphasic kinetics of glucose-stimulated insulin secretion. An early rapid and transient component (1st phase secretion) represents RRP release and a second slower and sustained component reflects a time- and ATP-dependent replenishment of

RRP by mobilization of granules from the reserve pool (for review, see ref. 3,34). Type-2 diabetes or non-insulin dependent diabetes mellitus (NIDDM) is associated with disturbances of this release pattern already at early stages of the disease displaying a characteristic lack of 1st phase secretion in response to an elevation of the glucose concentration.

Sulfonylureas are used in the treatment of NIDDM. Their principal effect is to stimulate insulin secretion from the beta-cells by their ability to inhibit the K_{ATP} channels in the beta-cell PM, which bypasses the physiological regulation of the channels by cytosolic concentrations of ATP and ADP.[35] The inhibition of K_{ATP} channels by sulfonylureas results in membrane depolarization, Ca^{2+} influx and insulin secretion as long as the drug is present.[32] It has recently been demonstrated that the K_{ATP} channel is composed of two components: a sulfonylurea receptor (SUR) - which similarly to MDR1 (ABCB1) and CFTR (ABCC7) belongs to the superfamily of ATP-binding cassette (ABC) transporters - and an inward-rectifying K^{+} channel protein ($K_{ir6.2}$) (for review, see ref. 36). The binding of sulfonylureas to the beta-cell isoform of SUR, SUR1 (ABCC8), leads to the closure of the K_{ATP} channel. It is intriguing, however, that more than 90% of the high-affinity sulfonylurea binding sites in the beta-cell are intracellular and appear to co-localize with the insulin-containing secretory granules.[37,38] The role and molecular identity of these intracellular sulfonylurea binding sites is not known, but it has been reported that sulfonylureas potentiate insulin secretion also by a direct effect on the exocytotic machinery.[39] This stimulation requires low extracellular glucose concentrations, depends on protein kinase C (PKC) and is observed at therapeutic concentrations of sulfonylureas. This is very much as described in pancreatic ZG membranes (see above). We therefore hypothesized that sulfonylurea-modulated channels could also be present in beta-cell granules and participate in sulfonylurea-induced stimulation of secretion.

3.1 A 65-kDa mdr1-Like Sulfonylurea-Binding Protein Regulates Exocytosis[40]

To elucidate the mechanisms underlying the direct stimulatory effect of sulfonylureas on the exocytotic machinery, we measured exocytosis under voltage clamp conditions, which circumvents sulfonylurea-mediated depolarization of the cell. Ca^{2+} and test substances were dialyzed into the intracellular space through the recording electrode. Exocytosis and discharge of granule contents were determined by combining cell capacitance measurements and amperometric detection of released serotonin.

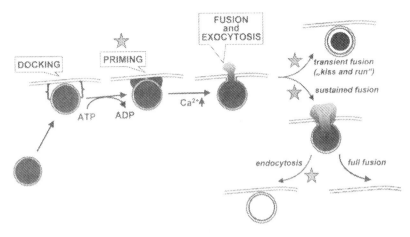

Figure 1. Modulation of Ca^{2+}-dependent exocytotic secretion by granule ion channels. Putative pre- and post-exocytotic processes affected by ion channels and their regulatory subunits are labelled by "stars". For further details, see text. The model is compiled and inspired from extensive reviews on exocytotic secretion in pancreatic acinar and beta cells.[2,12,31] To better illustrate the mechanisms of exocytotic secretion the granule contents, which consist of macromolecular matrix / secretory proteins as well as small anorganic / organic molecules, are represented by a black circle and a brownish ring, respectively.

Stimulation of exocytosis by the sulfonylurea tolbutamide was observed by a stepwise increase in $[Ca^{2+}]$ due to photorelease of caged Ca^{2+}. Pharmacologically, the exocytotic mechanism affected by tolbutamide was very similar to the beta-cell plasma membrane K_{ATP} channels, because it was inhibited by diazoxide but not by pinacidil, which activates cardiac/vascular K_{ATP} channels by binding to the SUR2A/B (ABCC9) sulfonylurea receptor.[41] Thus, the data indicated the involvement of a SUR1 (ABCC8)-like regulatory mechanism in beta-cell exocytosis. Evidence for a similar mechanism as in ZG, where a 65kDa mdr1 gene product confers the modulation by sulfonylureas (see above), was obtained in islet beta-cells.[40] Antibodies against cytosolic domains of ABCB1 (mdr1) (JSB-1 and C219) detected a protein of 65kDa in beta-cell granule membrane fractions. In addition, UV-cross-linking revealed binding of the sulfonylurea glibenclamide to a protein of about 65kDa in the granule fraction. Intracellular application of the ABCB1 antibody JSB-1 abolished the stimulatory action of sulfonylureas on exocytosis. Furthermore, a blocker of ABCB1, tamoxifen, prevented the stimulation of exocytosis induced by tolbutamide. Taken together, the data suggested that sulfonylureas bind to a granule membrane protein of 65kDa, which may be an ABCB1 (mdr1) gene product. This resulted in the activation of the exocytotic machinery. Because Ca^{2+}-dependent exocytosis induced by sulfonylureas was also inhibited by the Cl⁻ channel blocker DIDS,[40] we hypothesized that activation of the exocytotic machinery by sulfonylureas might also involve opening of Cl⁻ channels in the granule membrane.

3.2 A ClC-3 Cl⁻ channel provides the counterions for granule acidification driven by a vacuolar-type (V-type) H⁺-ATPase

We found that Ca^{2+}-dependent exocytosis in the presence or absence of tolbutamide was strongly inhibited by replacing intracellular Cl⁻ with glutamate.[42] In addition, antibodies against the chloride channel ClC-3 cross-reacted with beta-cell granules. Immunoblot analysis of beta-cell homogenates and a granule fraction revealed an immunoreactive band with a molecular weight of about 90kDa, as expected for the non-glycosylated form of ClC-3. When a functional antibody against the C-terminal cytosolic domain of ClC-3 was dialyzed into the intracellular space through the patch-clamp electrode, exocytosis was strongly inhibited. In contrast, a non-functional antibody against the N-terminal domain of ClC-3 was without effect.[42] We concluded that granule Cl⁻ flux carried by ClC-3 channels is required for Ca^{2+}-dependent exocytosis in beta-cells and hypothesized that acidification by electrogenic H⁺ pumping into the granule might require a shunt-conductance to prevent the build-up of an electrical potential, which would be provided by a ClC-3 Cl⁻ channel. Indeed, exocytosis was also prevented by bafilomycin A, which irreversibly blocks V-ATPases, or by addition of the protonophore CCCP, which abolishes pH gradients across membranes.[42] Granule acidification can be measured with the fluorescent acidotropic probe LysoSensor green, which accumulates in acidic compartments (mostly granules in beta-cells) as the result of protonation. Following intracellular dialysis with 3mM MgATP and 1.5μM Ca^{2+} through the patch-pipette, there was a net granular acidification. Acidification was prevented by inclusion of 100μM DIDS in the pipette solution. There was a strong decrease of fluorescence (i.e. an increase of pH) when the protonophore CCCP was introduced into the cytosol. We concluded that electrogenic Cl⁻ ion transport through ClC-3 provides the counterions required for H^+ flux across the granule membrane and thereby modulate the exocytotic capacity of the beta-cell.[42]

To determine at what stage exocytosis was modulated by granular Cl^- and H^+ fluxes, the kinetics of exocytosis elicited by trains of voltage-clamp depolarization were analyzed to provide an estimate of the rates of processes prior to exocytosis. Pancreatic beta-cells were maximally stimulated and the size of the RRP and the rate of its turnover were estimated by capacitance measurements. The experiments indicated that Cl^- fluxes mediated by ClC-3 are involved in the "priming" reaction of insulin granules for Ca^{2+}-elicited exocytosis.[42] Granule acidification driven by the H^+-pump and/or maintenance of a pH gradient, however, appeared to be necessary for the "priming" reaction of the RRP (Figure 1). A low granule pH seemed to be required for granules that are ready for exocytosis. Conversely, dissipation of a pH gradient might induce granule "de-priming" and prevent exocytosis. How would granular acidification affect the final steps of exocytosis? We speculated that a low granular pH could influence the exocytotic machinery by inducing conformational changes in SNARE proteins, rendering them more fusogenic.[43] This mechanism may differ in pancreatic acinar cells, where an acidic ZG pH is not requisite for exocytosis and protein secretion.[44]

4.   PERSPECTIVES

The identification of secretory granule ion channels and the characterization of their physiological significance during pre- and post-exocytotic events could gain importance for the development of therapeutic drugs controlling secretory events. This is particularly relevant because secretory granules, similarly as other intracellular organelles, seem to be equipped with specific sets of ion channels, which represent ideal targets for the development of drugs with high tissue and/or cell specificity and a selective mode of action. The use of putative drugs as activators or inhibitors of secretory granule ion channels could thus significantly contribute to the improvement of pathophysiological disease conditions, such as CF, acute pancreatic, or NIDDM.

ACKNOWLEDGMENTS

I thank Prof. Patrik Rorsman (Lund University, Sweden, and Oxford Centre for Diabetes, Endocrinology and Metabolism, UK) for his support and interest in my work. Funding in my laboratory was provided by the Deutsche Forschungsgemeinschaft, the Deutsche Mukoviszidose e.V., the

Novo Nordisk Foundation, and start-up funds from the University of Witten/Herdecke.

REFERENCES

1. R. Jahn, T. Lang, and T. C. Südhof, Membrane fusion, *Cell* **112,** 519-533 (2003).
2. S. Barg, C. S. Olofsson, J. Schriever-Abeln, A. Wendt, S. Gebre-Medhin, E. Renström, and P. Rorsman, Delay between fusion pore opening and peptide release from large dense-core vesicles in neuroendocrine cells, *Neuron* **33,** 287-299 (2002).
3. P. Rorsman and E. Renstrom, Insulin granule dynamics in pancreatic beta cells, *Diabetologia* **46,** 1029-1045 (2003).
4. R. D. Burgoyne and M. J. Clague, Calcium and calmodulin in membrane fusion, *Biochim. Biophys. Acta* **1641,** 137-143 (2003).
5. H. Y. Gaisano, M. Ghai, P. N. Malkus, L. Sheu, A. Bouquillon, M. K. Bennett, and W. S. Trimble, Distinct cellular locations of the syntaxin family of proteins in rat pancreatic acinar cells, *Mol. Biol. Cell* **7,** 2019-2027 (1996).
6. N. J. Hansen, W. Antonin, and J. M. Edwardson, Identification of SNAREs involved in regulated exocytosis in the pancreatic acinar cell, *J. Biol. Chem.* **274,** 22871-22876 (1999).
7. R. Kuver, J. H. Klinkspoor, W. R. Osborne, S. P. Lee, Mucous granule exocytosis and CFTR expression in gallbladder epithelium. *Glycobiology* **10,** 49-157 (2000).
8. C. R. Marino, L. M. Matovcik, F. S. Gorelick, and J. A. Cohn, Localization of the cystic fibrosis transmembrane conductance regulator in pancreas, *J. Clin. Invest.* **88,** 712-716 (1991).
9. M. K. Park, R. B. Lomax, A. V. Tepikin, and O. H. Petersen, Local uncaging of caged Ca^{2+} reveals distribution of Ca^{2+}-activated Cl⁻ channels in pancreatic acinar cells, *Proc. Natl. Acad. Sci. USA.* **98,** 10948-10953 (2001).
10. Y. Maruyama, G. Inooka, Y. K. Li, Y. Miyashita, and H. Kasai, Agonist-induced localized Ca^{2+} spikes directly triggering exocytotic secretion in exocrine pancreas, *EMBO J.* **12,** 3017-3022 (1993).
11. C. M. Fuller, L. Eckhardt, and I. Schulz, Ionic and osmotic dependence of secretion from permeabilised acini of the rat pancreas, *Pflügers Arch.* **413,** 385-394, (1989).
12. F. Thévenod, Ion channels in secretory granules of the pancreas and their role in exocytosis and release of secretory proteins, *Am. J. Physiol. Cell Physiol.* **283,** C651-C672 (2002).
13. F. Thévenod, K. V. Chathadi, B. Jiang, and U. Hopfer, ATP-sensitive K^+ conductance in pancreatic zymogen granules: block by glyburide and activation by diazoxide, *J. Membrane Biol.* **129,** 253-266 (1992).
14. F. Thévenod, I. Anderie, and I. Schulz, Monoclonal antibodies against MDR1 P-glycoprotein inhibit chloride conductance and label a 65-kDa protein in pancreatic zymogen granule membranes, *J. Biol. Chem.* **269,** 24410-24417 (1994).
15. F. Thévenod, J. P. Hildebrandt, J. Striessnig, H. R. de Jonge, and I. Schulz, Chloride and potassium conductances of mouse pancreatic zymogen granules are inversely regulated by a approximately 80-kDa *mdr1a* gene product, *J. Biol. Chem.* **271,** 3300-3305 (1996).
16. M. Braun, I. Anderie, and F. Thévenod, Evidence for a 65 kDa sulfonylurea receptor in rat pancreatic zymogen granule membranes, *FEBS Lett.* **411,** 255-259 (1997).
17. M. A. Carew and P. Thorn, Identification of ClC-2-like chloride currents in pig pancreatic acinar cells, *Pflügers Arch.* **433,** 84-90 (1996).

18. F. Thévenod, E. Roussa, D. J. Benos, and C. M. Fuller, Relationship between a HCO$_3^-$ - permeable conductance and a CLCA protein from rat pancreatic zymogen granule, *Biochem. Biophys. Res. Commun.* **300**, 546-554 (2003).

19. B. U. Pauli, M. Abdel-Ghany, H. C. Cheng, A. D. Gruber, H. A. Archibald, and R. C. Elble, Molecular characteristics and functional diversity of CLCA family members, *Clin. Exp. Pharmacol. Physiol.* **27**, 901-905 (2000).

20. C. M. Fuller, H. L. Ji, A. Tousson, R. C. Elble, B. U. Pauli, and D. J. Benos, Ca^{2+}-activated Cl$^-$ channels: a newly emerging anion transport family, *Pflügers Arch.* **443** (Suppl. 1), S107-S110 (2001).

21. I. Leverkoehne and A. D. Gruber, The murine mCLCA3 (alias gob-5) protein is located in the mucin granule membranes of intestinal, respiratory, and uterine goblet cells, *J. Histochem. Cytochem.* **50**, 829-838 (2002).

22. A. D. Gruber, R. Gandhi, and B. U. Pauli, The murine calcium-sensitive chloride channel (mCaCC) is widely expressed in secretory epithelia and in other select tissues, *Histochem. Cell Biol.* **110**, 43-49 (1998).

23. S. D. Freedman, H. F. Kern, and G. A. Scheele, Cleavage of GPI-anchored proteins from the plasma membrane activates apical endocytosis in pancreatic acinar cells, *Eur. J. Cell Biol.* **75**, 163-173 (1998).

24. B. R. Grubb and R. C. Boucher, Pathophysiology of gene-targeted mouse models for cystic fibrosis, *Physiol. Rev.* **79** (Suppl. 1), S193-S214 (1999).

25. M. Suzuki, K. Fujikura, K. Kotake, N. Inagaki, S. Seino, and K. Takata, Immunolocalization of sulphonylurea receptor 1 in rat pancreas, *Diabetologia* **42**, 1204-1211 (1999).

26. J. Robbins, KCNQ potassium channels: physiology, pathophysiology, and pharmacology, *Pharmacol. Ther.* **90**, 1-19 (2001).

27. R. Warth, M. Garcia Alzamora, J. K. Kim, A. Zdebik, R. Nitschke, M. Bleich, U. Gerlach, J. Barhanin, and S. J. Kim, The role of KCNQ1/KCNE1 K$^+$ channels in intestine and pancreas: lessons from the KCNE1 knockout mouse, *Pflügers Arch.* **443**, 822-828 (2002).

28. C. Lerche, G. Seebohm, C. I. Wagner, C. R. Scherer, L. Dehmelt, I. Abitbol, U. Gerlach, J. Brendel, B. Attali, and A.E. Busch, Molecular impact of MinK on the enantiospecific block of I$_{Ks}$ by chromanols, *Br. J. Pharmacol.* **131**, 1503-1506 (2000).

29. B. P. Jena, S. W. Schneider, J. P. Geibel, P. Webster, H. Oberleithner, and K. C. Sritharan, G$_i$ regulation of secretory vesicle swelling examined by atomic force microscopy, *Proc. Natl. Acad. Sci. USA* **94**, 13317-13322 (1997).

30. S. W. Schneider, K. C. Sritharan, J. P. Geibel, H. Oberleithner, and B. P. Jena, Surface dynamics in living acinar cells imaged by atomic force microscopy: identification of plasma membrane structures involved in exocytosis, *Proc. Natl. Acad. Sci. USA* **94**, 316-321 (1997).

31. S. W. Schneider, Kiss and run mechanism in exocytosis, *J. Membrane Biol.* **181**, 67-76 (2001).

32. F. M. Ashcroft, and P. Rorsman, Electrophysiology of the pancreatic beta-cell, *Prog. Biophys. Mol. Biol.* **54**, 87-143 (1989).

33. J. Lang, Molecular mechanisms and regulation of insulin exocytosis as a paradigm of endocrine secretion, *Eur. J. Biochem.* **259**, 3-17 (1999).

34. P. Rorsman, L. Eliasson, E. Renstrom, J. Gromada, S. Barg, and S. Göpel, The cell physiology of biphasic insulin secretion, *News Physiol. Sci.* **15**, 72-77 (2000).

35. S. J. Ashcroft, I. Niki, S. Kenna, L. Weng, J. Skeer, B. Coles, and F. M. Ashcroft, The beta-cell sulfonylurea receptor, *Adv. Exp. Med. Biol.* **334**, 47-61 (1993).

36. L. Aguilar-Bryan and J. Bryan, Molecular biology of adenosine triphosphate-sensitive potassium channels, *Endocr. Rev.* **20**, 101-135 (1999).
37. J. L. Carpentier, F. Sawano, M. Ravazzola, and W. J. Malaisse, Internalization of ^{3}H-glibenclamide in pancreatic islet cells, *Diabetologia* **29**, 259-261 (1986).
38. S. E. Ozanne, P. C. Guest, J. C. Hutton, and C. N. Hales, Intracellular localization and molecular heterogeneity of the sulphonylurea receptor in insulin-secreting cells, *Diabetologia* **38**, 277-282 (1995).
39. L. Eliasson, E. Renstrom, C. Ämmäla, P. O. Berggren, A. M. Bertorello, K. Bokvist, A. Chibalin, J. T. Deeney, P. R. Flatt, J. Gabel, J. Gromada, O. Larsson, P. Lindstrom, C. J. Rhodes, and P. Rorsman, PKC-dependent stimulation of exocytosis by sulfonylureas in pancreatic beta-cells, *Science* **271**, 813-815 (1996).
40. S. Barg, E. Renström, P.-O. Berggren, A. Bertorello, K. Bokvist, M. Braun, L. Eliasson, W. E. Holmes, M. Köhler, P. Rorsman, and F. Thévenod, The stimulatory action of tolbutamide on Ca^{2+}-dependent exocytosis in pancreatic □-cells is mediated by a 65 kDa mdr-like P-glycoprotein, *Proc. Natl. Acad. Sci. USA* **96**, 5539-5544 (1999).
41. T. Shindo, M. Yamada, S. Isomoto, Y. Horio, and Y. Kurachi, SUR2 subtype (A and B)-dependent differential activation of the cloned ATP-sensitive K^+ channels by pinacidil and nicorandil, *Br. J. Pharmacol.* **124**, 985-991 (1998).
42. S. Barg, P. Huang, L. Eliasson, D. J. Nelson, S. Obermüller, P. Rorsman, F. Thévenod, and E. Renström, Priming of insulin granules for exocytosis by granular Cl⁻ uptake and acidification, *J. Cell Sci.* **114**, 2145-2154 (2001).
43. R. B. Sutton, D. Fasshauer, R. Jahn, and A. T. Brunger, Crystal structure of a SNARE complex involved in synaptic exocytosis at 2.4 A resolution, *Nature* **395**, 347-353 (1998).
44. R. C. De Lisle, and J. A. Williams, Zymogen granule acidity is not required for stimulated pancreatic protein secretion, *Am. J. Physiol.* **253**, G711-G719 (1987).

Chapter 5

EPITHELIAL TRANSPORT AND INTRACELLULAR TRAFFICKING: PHYSIOLOGY AND PATHOPHYSIOLOGY

Helmut Kipp and Rolf K.H. Kinne
Max-Planck-Institut für molekulare Physiologie, Abteilung Epithelphysiologie, 44388 Dortmund, Germany. E-mail: helmut.kipp@mpi-dortmund.mpg.de

1.   INTRODUCTION

Transport proteins are frequently viewed as an integral, static component of the plasma membrane: They are synthesized inside the cell and then trafficked to the plasma membrane, where they stay until they are eventually degraded and substituted by newly synthesized transporters. However, the regulation of several membrane transporters is far more complex, since they are not only located in the plasma membrane but also in intracellular compartments. These intracellular compartments may be part of a regulatory mechanism: Membrane transporter may be shifted between the plasma membrane and intracellular sites, thereby regulating the amount of membrane transporters present at the cell surface. Utilizing this mechanism, the permeability of the plasma membrane for certain substrates can be rapidly increased or decreased allowing cells to quickly adapt to varying physiological conditions (i.e. substrate concentration) in their environment.

Over the course of the day, the amount of D-glucose to be reabsorbed varies in the small intestine. Immediately following a meal the amount of D-glucose to be absorbed is very high, whereas most of the time the amount is significantly lower. D-glucose is absorbed at the brush border membrane of the small intestine epithelium by the sodium/D-glucose cotransporter (SGLT1), which accumulates D-glucose in the epithelial cells powered by simultaneous down-hill transport of sodium. In the past we have studied the distribution of endogenous SGLT1 in Caco-2 cells, a cell culture model for human enterocytes, in order to identify SGLT1 populations, which might be part of a regulatory mechanism.[1]

2.   DISTRIBUTION OF SGLT1 IN CACO-2 CELLS

Using a set of newly developed epitope specific antibodies directed against loops of the SGLT1 protein, the cellular distribution of endogenous SGLT1 in Caco-2 cells was studied after biochemical cell fractionation (free flow electrophoresis) and by immunocytochemistry.

For subcellular fractionation of Caco-2 cells by free flow electrophoresis, a cellular organelle fraction was prepared from Caco-2 cells by gently disrupting the cells with nitrogen cavitation. Cellular organelles were then separated in an electric field and the obtained fractions were analyzed for endogenous and exogenous markers and for SGLT1 content (Figure 1). Apical and basolateral plasma membranes were identified by the activity of the marker enzymes alkaline phosphatase and sodium/potassium ATPase respectively (Figure 1A, D). Early and late endosomes were identified by the exogenous markers horseradish peroxydase and FITC-dextran (Figure 1B, E), which had been applied to the cells before the experiment according to a pulse-chase protocol. SGLT1 was identified in the fractions from the free flow electrophoresis by an ELISA assay using specific antibodies directed against SGLT1 (Figure 1C, F). Separation of cellular organelles was further enhanced by a gentle treatment of the COF with trypsin prior to free flow electrophoresis (Figure 1D, E, F). SGLT1 was detected not only in the apical plasma membrane, but also in intracellular compartments which co-purified after FFE separation with early endosomal factions. Interestingly, there was more SGLT1 detected in intracellular compartments than in the apical plasma membrane. The intracellular-apical SGLT1 distribution ratio was estimated by measurement of the areas below the respective curves of the ELISA assays; the intracellular-apical distribution ratio of SGLT1 was 2:1.

After separation of Caco-2 cell organelles by free flow electrophoresis, intracellular SGLT1 co-migrated with the so called endosomal fraction. However, this does not necessarily prove localization of SGLT1 to endosomes, since intracellular SGLT1 could also be located in organelles with properties comparable to endosomes during separation in an electric field. Actual evidence for endosomal SGLT1 was provided by immunocytochemical experiments.

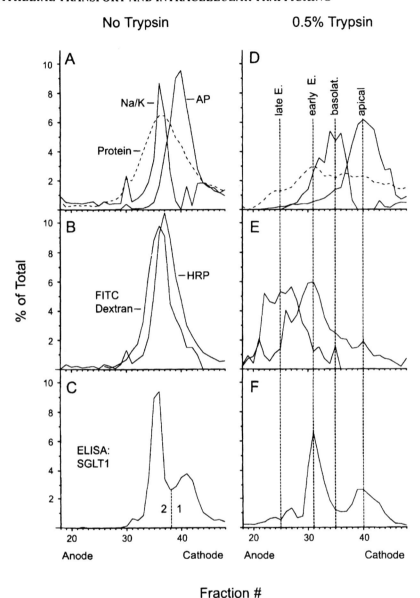

Figure 1. Analysis of SGLT1 distribution in Caco-2 cells by free flow electrophoresis (FFE). Fractions from the FFE were analyzed for the endogenous markers alkaline phosphatase (AP, apical plasma membrane), sodium/potassium ATPase (Na/K, basolateral membrane) and for the exogenous markers horseradish peroxydase (HRP, early endosomes) and FITC-dextran (late endosomes). SGLT1 was detected by an ELISA assay. Experiments were performed with and without prior treatment of the samples with trypsin. The figure is taken with permission from reference 1.

However, this does not necessarily prove localization of SGLT1 to endosomes, since intracellular SGLT1 could also be located in organelles with properties comparable to endosomes during separation in an electric field. Actual evidence for endosomal SGLT1 was provided by immunocytochemical experiments. Therefore, the cell surface of living Caco-2 cells were labeled with a fluorescent lipid or cell surface proteins were fluorescent-labeled with reactive biotin and streptavidin-Cy3. After incubation of the labeled cells at 37°C both fluorescent cell surface labels were taken up into the cell interior and were located in endosomes. Intracellular SGLT1 co-localized with the labeled endosomes indicating that intracellular SGLT1 actually resides in endosomes. Immuno-fluorescence microscopy further revealed that endosomes containing SGLT1 are associated with microtubules.

Intracellular populations of SGLT1 could represent transporters, which are on their journey from protein synthesis to the plasma membrane. However, intracellular SGLT1 compartments did not co-localize with organelles involved in the protein synthesis / degradation pathway (endoplasmatic reticulum, Golgi, lysosomes) after immunostaining of fixed Caco-2 cells. These results are in good agreement with our earlier observation that elimination of SGLT1 from the biosynthesis pathway with cycloheximide did not alter size nor shape of the intracellular SGLT1 population. Therefore, SGLT1 en route on the protein synthesis / degradation pathway contributes only to a very small extent to the total amount of SGLT1 present in the cell.

Although Caco-2 cells are a very common cell culture model for human enterocytes, Caco-2 cells were originally derived from a colon carcinoma. Regulation and distribution of SGLT1 might be different in a cancer cell compared to healthy tissue. We, therefore, investigated the distribution of SGLT1 in samples from human jejunum, which were obtained from the Pathology Department of a local hospital. Immunohistochemistry with SGLT1 specific antibodies of paraffin sections from human jejunum showed the major amount of SGLT1 inside absorptive cells, with a more prominent abundance at the apical pole of the cells. Only a faint staining of SGLT1 was observed in the brush border membrane. These observations resemble the results obtained in Caco-2 cells and highlight the validity of the Caco-2 cell model for the study of intracellular SGLT1 regulation in human enterocytes.

3.   DISTRIBUTION OF SGLT1 IN CACO-2 CELLS: THE STORY SO FAR

The distribution of SGLT1 in Caco-2 cells revealed so far is schematically presented in Figure 2. The amount of newly synthesized SGLT1 did not significantly contribute to the size of the total pool of SGLT1 present in Caco-2 cells. Assuming a steady state at which protein synthesis and protein degradation proceed at the same rate, only a small SGLT1 amount is added to and retrieved from a large existing SGLT1 pool in a given time interval. The large pool of SGLT1 is distributed between a SGLT1 population, which is located in the apical plasma membrane and a SGLT1 population, which is dispersed in intracellular, microtubule associated endosomes. The quantification of immuno-detectable SGLT1 in Caco-2 cells revealed a distribution ratio between apical plasma membrane and intracellular endosomes of 1:2. Most of the SGLT1 actually resides in intracellular endosomes, which are attached to microtubules! Since microtubules are the intracellular "railroad tracks", we assume that the endosomal pool of SGLT1 is highly mobile. We propose that SGLT1 can be shifted between the endosomal pool and the apical plasma membrane and that this is a mechanism by which D-glucose uptake into enterocytes can be regulated.

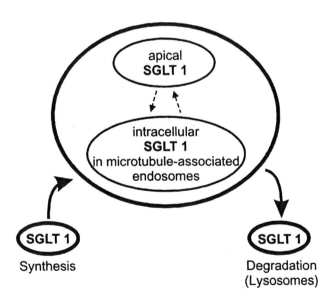

Figure 2. Tentative model for SGLT1 distribution in enterocytes cells. Dashed arrows indicate proposed regulation pathways for SGLT1 in enterocytes. See text for explanation.

4.   SYNOPSIS

Important for the normal physiological function of several membrane transporters is not only that they are expressed in a particular cell at all, moreover, the membrane transporter has to be trafficked at the appropriate time to the appropriate cellular location. Cystic fibrosis, the most frequent inherited disease in the white population, is caused by a mislead chloride channel, which is expressed in bronchial epithelial cells, but never attains the cell surface.[2] Inherited forms of intrahepatic cholestasis are due to mislead ATP binding cassette transporter, which are involved in bile formation in the canalicular membrane of hepatocytes.[3] The glucose-galactose malabsorption syndrome is caused by false intracellular sorting of SGLT1 in enterocytes.[4] Besides these examples there is a growing number of diseases, which were identified to be caused by deranged intracellular sorting of membrane transporters (trafficking diseases).[5,6] In several instances, point mutations in the genes for misguided membrane transporters have been identified, resulting in an exchange of a single amino acid in the transporter protein. However, the cascade of molecular events leading from a point mutation to false trafficking and ultimately to the full blown picture of the disease, is in all instances only poorly understood. Therefore, elucidation of the intracellular pathways and regulation of membrane transporters may help to understand the cause of trafficking diseases at a molecular level and provide clues for novel therapies.

REFERENCES

1. H. Kipp, S. Khoursandi, D. Scharlau, and R. K.-H. Kinne. More than apical: distribution of SGLT1 in Caco-2 cells. *Am. J. Physiol. Cell Physiol.* **285**, C737-C749 (2003).
2. R. R. Kopito. Biosynthesis and degradation of CFTR. *Physiol. Rev.* **79**, S167-S173 (1999).
3. H. Kipp and I. M. Arias. Trafficking of canalicular ABC transporters in hepatocytes. *Annu. Rev. Physiol.* **64**, 595-608 (2002).
4. E. M. Wright, E. Turk, and M. G. Martin. Molecular basis for glucose-galactose malabsorption. *Cell. Biochem. Biophys.* **36**, 115-121 (2002).
5. M. Aridor and L. A. Hannan. Traffic jam: a compendium of human diseases that affect intracellular transport processes. *Traffic* **1**, 836-851 (2000).
6. M. Aridor and L. A. Hannan. Traffic jams II: an update of diseases of intracellular transport. *Traffic* **3**, 781-790 (2002).

Chapter 6

KINASES, CELL VOLUME, AND THE REGULATION OF CHLORIDE CHANNELS

Florian Lang[1], Albrecht Lepple-Wienhues[1], Ildicko Szabo[1], Erich Gulbins[2], Monica Palmada[1], Sabine Wallisch[1], Christoph Böhmer[1], Karin Klingel[3] and Reinhard Kandolf[3]

[1]*Department of Physiology;* [2]*Department of Molecular Biology, University of Essen;* [3]*Department of Molecular Pathology, Eberhard-Karls-University of Tuebingen, Gmelinstrasse 5, D-72076 Tuebingen, Germany; Tel: +49 7071 29 72194; Fax: +49 7071 29 5618; e-mail: florian.lang@uni-tuebingen.de*

1. INTRODUCTION

The ability of cells to maintain constancy of their volume is one of the prerequisites of cell survival. Cell membranes are usually highly permeable to water which moves across the cell membranes according to the prevailing osmotic gradients.[1] Thus, to maintain a steady volume, the cells need to adjust the osmotic gradient across the cell membrane accordingly.

Upon cell shrinkage, cells have to increase cellular osmolarity that is achieved by accumulation of ions and organic osmolytes. The transport systems involved include the $Na^+,K^+,2Cl^-$ cotransporter and the Na^+/H^+ exchanger in parallel to the Cl^-/HCO_3^- exchanger. The latter tandem leads to gain of NaCl. The H^+ and HCO_3^- released are replenished from CO_2. Some cells activate Na^+ channels. The depolarization of the cell membrane drags Cl^- through Cl^- channels into the cell which parallels the entry of Na^+. Beyond that cells gain osmolarity by accumulative transport and/or intracellular generation of organic osmolytes, such as amino acids, taurine, inositol, betaine, sorbitol and glycerophosphorylcholine. Beyond modification of transport swollen cells further adapt their metabolism to decrease the osmotic load. Most importantly, cell swelling inhibits the degradation and favours the synthesis of proteins and glycogen. Thus, the

73

amino acids and glucose are incorporated into the osmotically less active macromolecules [2].

Upon cell swelling, cells have to reduce intracellular osmolarity, e.g. by activation of K^+ channels and/or Cl^- channels. The activity of the K^+ channels keeps the cell membrane hyperpolarized, which drives Cl^- exit. Some cells release K^+ and Cl^- via activation of a KCl symport. Organic osmolytes are released through Cl^- channels. Cell shrinkage stimulates the degradation of proteins and glycogen thus leading to the production of osmotically active amiono acids and glucose[2].

The cell volume regulatory mechanisms participate in the regulation a wide variety of cellular functions. For instance, the transcellular movement of solutes during epithelial transport is an ever changing challenge to cell volume constancy and cell volume regulatory mechanisms participate in the concerted tuning of solute entry and exit.[1,3-5] Cell volume influences neuronal excitability which depends on cell membrane potential and thus ion channel activity.[1,5] The influence of cell volume on metabolism impacts on the regulation of protein and glycogen metabolism. Insulin, for instance, increases hepatocyte volume by activation of $Na^+,K^+,2Cl^-$ cotransporter and the Na^+/H^+ exchanger , the resulting cell swelling subsequently inhibits the degradation and stimulates the synthesis of proteins and glycogen. Thus, cell swelling participates in the signaling of the antiproteolytic and antiglycogenolytic action of insulin.[2] Cell volume regulatory mechanisms participate in the machinery underlying migration which involves regulatory cell volume increase at the leading edge and regulatory cell volume decrease at the rear.[6] Among the prerequisites of cell proliferation is cell swelling [1,7] and one of the hallmarks of apoptotic cell death is cell shrinkage [1,8,9].

The molecular identity of the cell volume regulatory transport mechanisms is only partially known. Most importantly, the specific Cl^- channels involved are a matter of controversy. Similarly, the signalling mechanisms triggering Cl^- channel activity are poorly defined. In the following presentation, the role of two cell volume-sensitive kinases in the regulation of Cl^- channels will be discussed.

2.   LCK56 IN THE REGULATION OF ION CHANNELS

The lymphocyte Src-like kinase LCK56 is activated by cell swelling and inhibited by cell shrinkage.[10] The kinase activates the outwardly rectifying Cl^- channel ORCC.[10] Pharmacological inhibition or genetic knockout of LCK56 abrogates the activation of ORCC following cell swelling and subsequent regulatory cell volume decrease.[10] Purified LCK56 activates

ORCC even in the absence of cell swelling.[11] In lymphocytes from normal individuals, both cAMP and LCK56 activate ORCC.[12] ORCC in lymphocytes from CF patients is resistant to activation by cAMP but still activated by LCK56.[12] Triggering of the CD95 receptor or application of ceramide activates ORCC through LCK56, an effect required for subsequent apoptosis.[11]

The CD95 receptor triggers further results in LCK56-dependent inhibition of Na^+/H^+ exchange,[8] an effect again favouring cell shrinkage. However, inhibition of Na^+/H^+ exchange is slow and probably not due to direct phosphorylation by LCK56, which is activated within a few minutes following CD95 triggering.[13] Rather, Na^+/H^+ exchange activity may be secondary to ATP depletion.[8] The activation of ORCC and the inhibition of Na^+/H^+ exchange do not only shrink the cells but induce cytosolic acidification,[8] which may favour DNA fragmentation.[14]

CD95 receptor triggering has further been shown to result in an early inhibition of Kv1.3 K^+ channels,[13,15] the cell volume regulatory K^+ channels of Jurkat lymphocytes[16]. The effect requires LCK56 [13,17] and seems to be involved in the initiation of cell death via CD95. A late activation of Kv1.3 seems to support cell shrinkage in the execution phase of apoptosis suggesting a dual role of Kv1.3 in apoptosis.[18]

CD95 triggering further leads to inhibition of Ca^{2+} release activated Ca^{2+} channels (I_{CRAC}) which may be important in preventing activation of the cells rather than inducing apoptosis.[19]

With considerable delay, CD95 triggering leads to LCK56 independent release of the osmolyte taurine and presumably other organic osmolytes,[20, 21] an effect again supporting cell shrinkage.

3.   SERUM AND GLUCOCORTICOID INDUCIBLE KINASE AND THE REGULATION OF CL⁻ AND NA⁺ CHANNELS

The second cell volume-sensitive kinase regulating Cl⁻ channels is the serum and glucocorticoid inducible kinase SGK1. SGK1 was originally cloned as an early gene, induced by serum and glucocorticoids in rat mammary tumour cells.[22,23] The human isoform has been identified as a cell volume regulated-gene, transcriptionally upregulated by cell shrinkage.[24-27] Further stimulators of SGK1 transcription include mineralocorticoids,[28-32] gonadotropins,[33,34] tumour growth factor TGFß,[8,35,36] fibroblast growth factor FGF and platelet-derived growth factor PDGF[37] as well as other cytokines.[30,38]

To become functional, SGK1 requires activation by phosphorylation, through a signaling cascade including phosphatidylinositol (PI) 3-kinase and phosphoinositide dependent kinase PDK1 and PDK2.[39,40] The stimulators of SGK1 include insulin, insulin like growth factor, IGF1, and oxidation.[25,39]

Heterologous expression studies in *Xenopus* oocytes revealed the ability of SGK1 to activate the cystic fibrosis transmembrane regulator CFTR channel.[41] Given the marked upregulation of SGK1 in inflammatory lung disease[41, 42] this effect could participate in the stimulation of bronchial Cl⁻ secretion.

The potent transcriptional regulation of SGK1 by mineralocorticoids[28-32] is suggestive of a role of this kinase in the control of epithelial Na⁺ transport. A key channel in the mineralocorticoid regulation of renal tubular Na⁺ reabsorption is the epithelial Na⁺ channel ENaC.[43,44] As amplified elsewhere,[45] SGK1 indeed interacts with ENaC[46] and co-expression of SGK1 indeed markedly enhances the activity of ENaC, heterologously expressed in *Xenopus* oocytes.[8,29,31,41,47,48] SGK1 interacts with ENaC, not by direct phosphorylation of the channel protein,[8] but by inactivating the ubiquitin ligase Nedd4-2 (ref.[49,50]), which otherwise ubiquitinates ENaC thus preparing the channel protein for clearance from the cell membrane.[51] As a result, SGK1 increases the abundance of ENaC channel protein within the cell membrane.[47, 52] The functional relevance of ENaC regulation by SGK1 is illustrated by experiments in the SGK1 knockout (*sgk1-/-*) mouse.[53] Under normal supply of NaCl, the NaCl excretion of the *sgk1-/-* mouse is virtually identical to the NaCl excretion of wild type littermates (*sgk1+/+*). A NaCl deficient diet, however, discloses the impaired ability of the sgk1-/- mouse to lower renal Na⁺ output. Even though NaCl excretion decreases substantially under NaCl depletion in both, *sgk1-/-* and *sgk1+/+* mice, the renal NaCl loss remains significantly larger in *sgk1-/-* mice than in *sgk1+/+* mice, despite exaggerated increase of plasma aldosterone concentrations, decreased blood pressure, decrease in glomerular filtration rate and enhanced proximal tubular Na⁺ reabsorption in the *sgk1-/-* mice.[53] The phenotype of the *sgk1-/-* mouse is by far less severe than the phenotype of the ENaC knockout mouse[54] and the mineralocorticoid receptor knockout mouse.[55] Thus, renal ENaC function and renal mineralocorticoid action are partially but not completely dependent on the presence of SGK1. SGK1 probably further contributes to the regulation of renal Na⁺ excretion by insulin and IGF-1.[46,56,57]

The effects of SGK1 are not restricted to epithelial Cl⁻ and Na⁺ channels. Instead, the kinase regulates a wide variety of channels and transporters including the Na⁺/H⁺ exchanger NHE3,[58-60] the renal outer medullary K⁺ channel ROMK1,[61-63] the voltage-gated Na⁺ channel SCN5A,[64] the voltage-gated K⁺ channel KCNE1/KCNQ1,[65] the voltage-gated K⁺ channel

Kv1.3,[42,66,67] the $Na^+,K^+,2Cl^-$ cotransporter,[68] the glutamine transporter SN1,[69] the glutamate transporter EAAT1,[70] and the Na^+/K^+-ATPase.[71,72]

ACKNOWLEDGEMENTS

Research of the authors was supported by the Deutsche Forschungsgemeinschaft La 315/4-3, La 315/6-1, and La 315/11-1.

REFERENCES

1. F. Lang, G. L. Busch, M. Ritter, H. Volkl, S. Waldegger, E. Gulbins, and D. Haussinger, Functional significance of cell volume regulatory mechanisms, *Physiol. Rev.* **78**, 247-306 (1998).
2. D. Haussinger and F. Lang, Cell volume in the regulation of hepatic function: a mechanism for metabolic control, *Biochim. Biophys. Acta.* **1071**, 331-350 (1991).
3. F. Lang, G. Messner, and W. Rehwald, Electrophysiology of sodium-coupled transport in proximal renal tubules, *Am. J. Physiol.* **250**, F953-F962 (1986).
4. S. G. Schultz, Homocellular regulatory mechanisms in sodium-transporting epithelia: avoidance of extinction by "flush-through", *Am. J. Physiol.* **241**, F579-F590 (1981).
5. Wehner F. Cell Volume: sensors, regulators and functional significance. *Cell. Physiol. Biochem.* **Vol.** ed. Basel: Karger Verlag, 2000.
6. S. Grinstein, Ion exchangers in the regulation of cell volume and motility, *Proceedings of the IUPS* (2001).
7. M. Ritter and E. Woell, Modification of cellular ion transport by the Ha-ras oncogene: steps towards malignant transformation, *Cell. Physiol. Biochem.* **6**, 245-270 (1996).
8. F. Lang, J. Madlung, J. Bock, U. Lukewille, S. Kaltenbach, K. S. Lang, C. Belka, C. A. Wagner, H. J. Lang, E. Gulbins, and A. Lepple-Wienhues, Inhibition of Jurkat-T-lymphocyte Na+/H+-exchanger by CD95(Fas/Apo-1)-receptor stimulation, *Pflugers Arch.* **440**, 902-907 (2000).
9. J. Moran, X. Hernandez-Pech, H. Merchant-Larios, and H. Pasantes-Morales, Release of taurine in apoptotic cerebellar granule neurons in culture, *Pflugers Arch.* **439**, 271-277 (2000).
10. A. Lepple-Wienhues, I. Szabo, T. Laun, N. K. Kaba, E. Gulbins, and F. Lang, The tyrosine kinase p56lck mediates activation of swelling-induced chloride channels in lymphocytes, *J. Cell Biol.* **141**, 281-286 (1998).
11. I. Szabo, A. Lepple-Wienhues, K. N. Kaba, M. Zoratti, E. Gulbins, and F. Lang, Tyrosine kinase-dependent activation of a chloride channel in CD95-induced apoptosis in T lymphocytes, *Proc. Natl. Acad. Sci. U.S.A.* **95**, 6169-6174 (1998).
12. A. Lepple-Wienhues, U. Wieland, T. Laun, L. Heil, M. Stern, and F. Lang, A src-like kinase activates outwardly rectifying chloride channels in CFTR-defective lymphocytes, *FASEB J.* **15**, 927-931 (2001).
13. I. Szabo, E. Gulbins, H. Apfel, X. Zhang, P. Barth, A. E. Busch, K. Schlottmann, O. Pongs, and F. Lang, Tyrosine phosphorylation-dependent suppression of a voltage-gated K+ channel in T lymphocytes upon Fas stimulation, *J. Biol. Chem.* **271**, 20465-20469 (1996).

14. L. D. Shrode, H. Tapper, and S. Grinstein, Role of intracellular pH in proliferation, transformation, and apoptosis, *J. Bioenerg. Biomembr.* **29**, 393-399 (1997).

15. I. Szabo, E. Gulbins, and F. Lang, Regulation of Kv1.3 during Fas-induced apoptosis, *Cell. Physiol. Biochem.* **7**, 148-158 (1997).

16. C. Deutsch and L. Q. Chen, Heterologous expression of specific K+ channels in T lymphocytes: functional consequences for volume regulation, *Proc. Natl. Acad. Sci. U.S.A.* **90**, 10036-10040 (1993).

17. E. Gulbins, I. Szabo, K. Baltzer, and F. Lang, Ceramide-induced inhibition of T lymphocyte voltage-gated potassium channel is mediated by tyrosine kinases, *Proc. Natl. Acad. Sci. U.S.A.* **94**, 7661-7666 (1997).

18. N. M. Storey, M. Gomez-Angelats, C. D. Bortner, D. L. Armstrong, and J. A. Cidlowski, Stimulation of Kv1.3 potassium channels by death receptors during apoptosis in Jurkat T lymphocytes, *J. Biol. Chem.* **278**, 33319-33326 (2003).

19. A. Lepple-Wienhues, C. Belka, T. Laun, A. Jekle, B. Walter, U. Wieland, M. Welz, L. Heil, J. Kun, G. Busch, M. Weller, M. Bamberg, E. Gulbins, and F. Lang, Stimulation of CD95 (Fas) blocks T lymphocyte calcium channels through sphingomyelinase and sphingolipids, *Proc. Natl. Acad. Sci. U.S.A.* **96**, 13795-13800 (1999).

20. F. Lang, A. Lepple-Wienhues, M. Paulmichl, I. Szabo, D. Siemen, and E. Gulbins, Ion channels, cell volume, and apoptotic cell death, *Cell. Physiol. Biochem.* **8**, 285-92 (1998).

21. F. Lang, J. Madlung, D. Siemen, C. Ellory, A. Lepple-Wienhues, and E. Gulbins, The involvement of caspases in the CD95(Fas/Apo-1)- but not swelling-induced cellular taurine release from Jurkat T-lymphocytes, *Pflugers Arch.* **440**, 93-99 (2000).

22. M. K. Webster, L. Goya, and G. L. Firestone, Immediate-early transcriptional regulation and rapid mRNA turnover of a putative serine/threonine protein kinase, *J. Biol. Chem.* **268**, 11482-11485 (1993).

23. M. K. Webster, L. Goya, Y. Ge, A. C. Maiyar, and G. L. Firestone, Characterization of sgk, a novel member of the serine/threonine protein kinase gene family which is transcriptionally induced by glucocorticoids and serum, *Mol. Cell Biol.* **13**, 2031-2040 (1993).

24. L. M. Bell, M. L. Leong, B. Kim, E. Wang, J. Park, B. A. Hemmings, and G. L. Firestone, Hyperosmotic stress stimulates promoter activity and regulates cellular utilization of the serum- and glucocorticoid-inducible protein kinase (Sgk) by a p38 MAPK-dependent pathway, *J. Biol. Chem.* **275**, 25262-25272 (2000).

25. S. Waldegger, P. Barth, G. Raber, and F. Lang, Cloning and characterization of a putative human serine/threonine protein kinase transcriptionally modified during anisotonic and isotonic alterations of cell volume, *Proc. Natl. Acad. Sci. U.S.A.* **94**, 4440-4445 (1997).

26. S. Waldegger, M. Erdel, U. O. Nagl, P. Barth, G. Raber, S. Steuer, G. Utermann, M. Paulmichl, and F. Lang, Genomic organization and chromosomal localization of the human SGK protein kinase gene, *Genomics* **51**, 299-302 (1998).

27. S. Waldegger, S. Gabrysch, P. Barth, S. Fillon, and F. Lang, h-sgk serine-threonine protein kinase as transcriptional target of p38/MAP kinase pathway in HepG2 human hepatoma cells, *Cell. Physiol. Biochem.* **10**, 203-208 (2000).

28. F. E. Brennan and P. J. Fuller, Rapid upregulation of serum and glucocorticoid-regulated kinase (sgk) gene expression by corticosteroids in vivo, *Mol. Cell. Endocrinol.* **166**, 129-136 (2000).

29. S. Y. Chen, A. Bhargava, L. Mastroberardino, O. C. Meijer, J. Wang, P. Buse, G. L. Firestone, F. Verrey, and D. Pearce, Epithelial sodium channel regulated by aldosterone-induced protein sgk, *Proc. Natl. Acad. Sci. U.S.A.* **96**, 2514-2519 (1999).

30. R. T. Cowling and H. C. Birnboim, Expression of serum- and glucocorticoid-regulated kinase (sgk) mRNA is up-regulated by GM-CSF and other proinflammatory mediators in human granulocytes, *J. Leukoc. Biol.* **67**, 240-248 (2000).

31. A. Naray-Fejes-Toth, C. Canessa, E. S. Cleaveland, G. Aldrich, and G. Fejes-Toth, Sgk is an aldosterone-induced kinase in the renal collecting duct. Effects on epithelial Na^+ channels, *J. Biol. Chem.* **274**, 16973-16978 (1999).

32. A. Shigaev, C. Asher, H. Latter, H. Garty, and E. Reuveny, Regulation of sgk by aldosterone and its effects on the epithelial $Na(+)$ channel, *Am. J. Physiol. Renal Physiol.* **278**, F613-F619 (2000).

33. I. J. Gonzalez-Robayna, A. E. Falender, S. Ochsner, G. L. Firestone, and J. S. Richards, Follicle-Stimulating hormone (FSH) stimulates phosphorylation and activation of protein kinase B (PKB/Akt) and serum and glucocorticoid-Induced kinase (Sgk): evidence for A kinase-independent signaling by FSH in granulosa cells, *Mol. Endocrinol.* **14**, 1283-1300 (2000).

34. J. S. Richards, S. L. Fitzpatrick, J. W. Clemens, J. K. Morris, T. Alliston, and J. Sirois, Ovarian cell differentiation: a cascade of multiple hormones, cellular signals, and regulated genes, *Recent Prog. Horm. Res.* **50**, 223-254 (1995).

35. J. M. Kumar, D. P. Brooks, B. A. Olson, and N. J. Laping, Sgk, a putative serine/threonine kinase, is differentially expressed in the kidney of diabetic mice and humans, *J. Am. Soc. Nephrol.* **10**, 2488-2494 (1999).

36. S. Waldegger, K. Klingel, P. Barth, M. Sauter, M. L. Rfer, R. Kandolf, and F. Lang, h-sgk serine-threonine protein kinase gene as transcriptional target of transforming growth factor beta in human intestine, *Gastroenterology* **116**, 1081-1088 (1999).

37. S. P. Davies, H. Reddy, M. Caivano, and P. Cohen, Specificity and mechanism of action of some commonly used protein kinase inhibitors, *Biochem. J.* **351**, 95-105 (2000).

38. F. Lang and P. Cohen, Regulation and physiological roles of serum- and glucocorticoid-induced protein kinase isoforms, *Sci. STKE* **2001**, RE17 (2001).

39. T. Kobayashi and P. Cohen, Activation of serum- and glucocorticoid-regulated protein kinase by agonists that activate phosphatidylinositide 3-kinase is mediated by 3-phosphoinositide-dependent protein kinase-1 (PDK1) and PDK2, *Biochem. J.* **339**, 319-328 (1999).

40. J. Park, M. L. Leong, P. Buse, A. C. Maiyar, G. L. Firestone, and B. A. Hemmings, Serum and glucocorticoid-inducible kinase (SGK) is a target of the PI 3-kinase-stimulated signaling pathway, *EMBO J.* **18**, 3024-3033 (1999).

41. C. A. Wagner, M. Ott, K. Klingel, S. Beck, J. Melzig, B. Friedrich, K. N. Wild, S. Broer, I. Moschen, A. Albers, S. Waldegger, B. Tummler, M. E. Egan, J. P. Geibel, R. Kandolf, and F. Lang, Effects of the serine/threonine kinase SGK1 on the epithelial $Na(+)$ channel (ENaC) and CFTR: implications for cystic fibrosis, *Cell. Physiol. Biochem.* **11**, 209-218 (2001).

42. S. Wärntges, B. Friedrich, G. Henke, C. Duranton, P. A. Lang, S. Waldegger, R. Meyermann, D. Kuhl, E. J. Speckmann, N. Obermuller, R. Witzgall, A. F. Mack, H. J. Wagner, A. Wagner, S. Broer, and F. Lang, Cerebral localization and regulation of the cell volume-sensitive serum- and glucocorticoid-dependent kinase SGK1, *Pflugers Arch.* **443**, 617-624 (2002).

43. C. M. Canessa, J. D. Horisberger, and B. C. Rossier, Epithelial sodium channel related to proteins involved in neurodegeneration, *Nature* **361**, 467-470 (1993).

44. J. Loffing, M. Zecevic, E. Feraille, B. Kaissling, C. Asher, B. C. Rossier, G. L. Firestone, D. Pearce, and F. Verrey, Aldosterone induces rapid apical translocation of ENaC in early

portion of renal collecting system: possible role of SGK, *Am. J. Physiol. Renal Physiol.* **280**, F675-F682 (2001).

45. F. Verrey, J. Loffing, M. Zecevic, D. Heitzmann, and O. Staub, SGK1: aldosterone-induced relay of Na^+ transport regulation in distal kidney nephron cells, *Cell. Physiol. Biochem.* **13**, 021-028 (2003).

46. J. Wang, P. Barbry, A. C. Maiyar, D. J. Rozansky, A. Bhargava, M. Leong, G. L. Firestone, and D. Pearce, SGK integrates insulin and mineralocorticoid regulation of epithelial sodium transport, *Am. J. Physiol. Renal Physiol.* **280**, F303-F313 (2001).

47. D. Alvarez de la Rosa, P. Zhang, A. Naray-Fejes-Toth, G. Fejes-Toth, and C. M. Canessa, The serum and glucocorticoid kinase sgk increases the abundance of epithelial sodium channels in the plasma membrane of Xenopus oocytes, *J. Biol. Chem.* **274**, 37834-37839 (1999).

48. C. Böhmer, C. A. Wagner, S. Beck, I. Moschen, J. Melzig, A. Werner, J. T. Lin, F. Lang, and F. Wehner, The shrinkage-activated Na(+) conductance of rat hepatocytes and its possible correlation to rENaC, *Cell. Physiol. Biochem.* **10**, 187-194 (2000).

49. C. Debonneville, S. Y. Flores, E. Kamynina, P. J. Plant, C. Tauxe, M. A. Thomas, C. Munster, A. Chraibi, J. H. Pratt, J. D. Horisberger, D. Pearce, J. Loffing, and O. Staub, Phosphorylation of Nedd4-2 by Sgk1 regulates epithelial Na(+) channel cell surface expression, *EMBO J.* **20**, 7052-7059 (2001).

50. P. M. Snyder, D. R. Olson, and B. C. Thomas, Serum and glucocorticoid-regulated kinase modulates Nedd4-2-mediated inhibition of the epithelial Na+ channel, *J. Biol. Chem.* **277**, 5-8 (2002).

51. O. Staub, I. Gautschi, T. Ishikawa, K. Breitschopf, A. Ciechanover, L. Schild, and D. Rotin, Regulation of stability and function of the epithelial Na+ channel (ENaC) by ubiquitination, *EMBO J.* **16**, 6325-6336 (1997).

52. C. A. Wagner, B. Friedrich, I. Setiawan, F. Lang, and S. Broer, The use of Xenopus laevis oocytes for the functional characterization of heterologously expressed membrane proteins, *Cell. Physiol. Biochem.* **10**, 1-12 (2000).

53. P. Wulff, V. Vallon, D. Y. Huang, H. Volkl, F. Yu, K. Richter, M. Jansen, M. Schlunz, K. Klingel, J. Loffing, G. Kauselmann, M. R. Bosl, F. Lang, and D. Kuhl, Impaired renal Na(+) retention in the sgk1-knockout mouse, *J. Clin. Invest.* **110**, 1263-1268 (2002).

54. E. Hummler, P. Barker, J. Gatzy, F. Beermann, C. Verdumo, A. Schmidt, R. Boucher, and B. C. Rossier, Early death due to defective neonatal lung liquid clearance in alpha-ENaC-deficient mice, *Nat. Genet.* **12**, 325-328 (1996).

55. S. Berger, M. Bleich, W. Schmid, T. J. Cole, J. Peters, H. Watanabe, W. Kriz, R. Warth, R. Greger, and G. Schutz, Mineralocorticoid receptor knockout mice: pathophysiology of Na+ metabolism, *Proc. Natl. Acad. Sci. U.S.A.* **95**, 9424-9429 (1998).

56. B. L. Blazer-Yost, X. Liu, and S. I. Helman, Hormonal regulation of ENaCs: insulin and aldosterone, *Am. J. Physiol.* **274**, C1373-C1379 (1998).

57. B. L. Blazer-Yost, T. G. Paunescu, S. I. Helman, K. D. Lee, and C. J. Vlahos, Phosphoinositide 3-kinase is required for aldosterone-regulated sodium reabsorption, *Am. J. Physiol.* **277**, C531-C536 (1999).

58. G. L. Firestone, J. R. Giampaolo, and B. A. O'Keeffe, Stimulus-dependent regulation of the serum and glucocorticoid inducible protein kinase (Sgk) transcription, subcellular localization and enzymatic activity, *Cell. Physiol. Biochem.* **13**, 1-12 (2003).

59. C. C. Yun, Y. Chen, and F. Lang, Glucocorticoid activation of Na(+)/H(+) exchanger isoform 3 revisited. The roles of SGK1 and NHERF2, *J. Biol. Chem.* **277**, 7676-7683 (2002).

60. C. C. Yun, Concerted Roles of SGK1 and the Na$^+$/H$^+$ Exchanger Regulatory Factor 2 (NHERF2) in Regulation of NHE3, *Cell. Physiol. Biochem.* **13**, 029-040 (2003).
61. M. Palmada, H. M. Embark, C. Yun, C. Bohmer, and F. Lang, Molecular requirements for the regulation of the renal outer medullary K(+) channel ROMK1 by the serum- and glucocorticoid-inducible kinase SGK1, *Biochem. Biophys. Res. Commun.* **311**, 629-634 (2003).
62. M. Palmada, H. M. Embark, A. W. Wyatt, C. Bohmer, and F. Lang, Negative charge at the consensus sequence for the serum- and glucocorticoid-inducible kinase, SGK1, determines pH sensitivity of the renal outer medullary K+ channel, ROMK1, *Biochem. Biophys. Res. Commun.* **307**, 967-972 (2003).
63. C. C. Yun, M. Palmada, H. M. Embark, O. Fedorenko, Y. Feng, G. Henke, I. Setiawan, C. Boehmer, E. J. Weinman, S. Sandrasagra, C. Korbmacher, P. Cohen, D. Pearce, and F. Lang, The Serum and Glucocorticoid-Inducible Kinase SGK1 and the Na(+)/H(+) Exchange Regulating Factor NHERF2 Synergize to Stimulate the Renal Outer Medullary K(+) Channel ROMK1, *J. Am. Soc. Nephrol.* **13**, 2823-2830 (2002).
64. C. Boehmer, V. Wilhelm, M. Palmada, S. Wallisch, G. Henke, H. Brinkmeier, P. Cohen, B. Pieske, and F. Lang, Serum and glucocorticoid inducible kinases in the regulation of the cardiac sodium channel SCN5A, *Cardiovasc. Res.* **57**, 1079-1084 (2003).
65. H. M. Embark, C. Bohmer, V. Vallon, F. Luft, and F. Lang, Regulation of KCNE1-dependent K(+) current by the serum and glucocorticoid-inducible kinase (SGK) isoforms, *Pflugers Arch.* **445**, 601-606 (2003).
66. N. Gamper, S. Fillon, S. M. Huber, Y. Feng, T. Kobayashi, P. Cohen, and F. Lang, IGF-1 up-regulates K+ channels via PI3-kinase, PDK1 and SGK1, *Pflugers Arch.* **443**, 625-634 (2002).
67. N. Gamper, S. Fillon, Y. Feng, B. Friedrich, P. A. Lang, G. Henke, S. M. Huber, T. Kobayashi, P. Cohen, and F. Lang, K(+) channel activation by all three isoforms of s, *Pflugers Arch.* **445**, 60-66 (2002).
68. F. Lang, K. Klingel, C. A. Wagner, C. Stegen, S. Warntges, B. Friedrich, M. Lanzendorfer, J. Melzig, I. Moschen, S. Steuer, S. Waldegger, M. Sauter, M. Paulmichl, V. Gerke, T. Risler, G. Gamba, G. Capasso, R. Kandolf, S. C. Hebert, S. G. Massry, and S. Broer, Deranged transcriptional regulation of cell-volume-sensitive kinase hSGK in diabetic nephropathy, *Proc. Natl. Acad. Sci. U.S.A.* **97**, 8157-8162 (2000).
69. C. Boehmer, F. Okur, I. Setiawan, S. Broer, and F. Lang, Properties and regulation of glutamine transporter SN1 by protein kinases SGK and PKB, *Biochem. Biophys. Res. Commun.* **306**, 156-162 (2003).
70. C. Boehmer, G. Henke, R. Schniepp, M. Palmada, J. D. Rothstein, S. Broer, and F. Lang, Regulation of the glutamate transporter EAAT1 by the ubiquitin ligase Nedd4-2 and the serum and glucocorticoid-inducible kinase isoforms SGK1/3 and protein kinase B, *J. Neurochem.* **86**, 1181-1188 (2003).
71. G. Henke, I. Setiawan, C. Bohmer, and F. Lang, Activation of Na(+)/K(+)-ATPase by the Serum and Glucocorticoid-Dependent Kinase Isoforms, *Kidney Blood Press. Res.* **25**, 370-374 (2002).
72. I. Setiawan, G. Henke, Y. Feng, C. Bohmer, L. A. Vasilets, W. Schwarz, and F. Lang, Stimulation of Xenopus oocyte Na(+),K(+)ATPase by the serum and glucocorticoid-dependent kinase sgk1, *Pflugers Arch.* **444**, 426-431 (2002).

Chapter 7

THE CLCAS: PROTEINS WITH ION CHANNEL, CELL ADHESION AND TUMOR SUPPRESSOR FUNCTIONS

Catherine M. Fuller, Gergely Kovacs, Susan J. Anderson, and Dale J. Benos
Dept. of Physiology and Biophysics,University of Alabama at Birmingham, 1918 University Boulevard, Birmingham, AL 35294 USA. Tel: (205) 934-6227. Email: fuller@physiology.uab.edu

1.   INTRODUCTION

Calcium-activated chloride currents have been recorded from nearly every cell type. However, while there are some features common to these currents from all cells, the multiplicity of anion current, conductance, and channel footprints associated with increases in cell calcium, combined with the lack of suitable high-affinity pharmacological probes and general paucity of molecular information, have made it difficult to assign any one conductance to any one channel. Despite this, several possible candidates for the role of CaCC have arisen in recent years including ClC3,[1] and more recently the bestrophins,[2-4] proteins originally associated with a form of macular dystrophy. We have focused on a family of proteins termed the CLCAs. These studies originated with a quest for the then unknown Cl⁻ channel underlying the CF defect. Using classical biochemical techniques, Ran and colleagues identified a protein from apical membrane vesicles of bovine trachea that when reconstituted into artificial liposomes was associated with DIDS-sensitive I^{125} uptake.[5,6] This material was separated by SDS-PAGE and an antibody raised to a 38 kDa polypeptide that represented the major band present. When this antibody was used in the further immunopurfication of solubulized tracheal membranes, the eluted protein resulted in a 260-fold enhancement in DIDS-sensitive I^{125} uptake as compared to the unpurified material.[6] The antibody decorated the apical membrane of the bovine trachea and reconstitution of this immunopurified material into planar lipid bilayers was associated with the appearance of an anion channel with an I> Cl selectivity profile and a DIDS-sensitive single channel conductance of ~ 25 pS in symmetrical 100 mM KCl solutions.[7] When examined by SDS-PAGE and immunoblotting, the immunopurified material migrated at approximately 140 kDa. The chance observation that after prolonged storage at -80°C, channel activity could no longer be detected in the bilayer system and that this was associated with loss of the 140 kDa band and appearance of the 38 kDa band, led us to propose that the channel protein was a homomultimer and was sensitive to reduction. The finding that the chemical reducing agent DTT also abolished channel activity was consistent with this interpretation.[7] Channel activity was sensitive to Ca^{2+}, but not *that* sensitive; the concentration of Ca^{2+} in the bath needed to be elevated to between 5-10 μM in order to see a significant increase in channel open probability (P_o). Further studies revealed that the sensitivity of the immunopurified channel to Ca^{2+} could be greatly increased by addition of multifunctional CaMK II (+ ATP and calmodulin), and that the protein could be directly phosphorylated by CaMK II.[8] This maneuver shifted the dose-response curve for Ca^{2+} to the left, such that peak channel opening was now seen between 0.5-1 μM [Ca^{2+}].

Using the same polyclonal antibody to screen a tracheal expression library as was used to immunopurify the protein from tracheal membrane vesicles, led us to identify a cDNA that coded for a protein of 903 amino acids currently termed bCLCA1.[9] The translated protein sequence also contained several consensus phosphorylation sites for multifunctional CaMK II and PKC. In addition, several sites for N-linked glycosylation sites were predicted, as were four transmembrane domains. The corresponding cRNA was expressed in Xenopus oocytes and was associated with a large outwardly rectified Cl current that was activated by Ca^{2+}. It was possible to express the clone in oocytes, because we took advantage of the sensitivity of the endogenous Ca^{2+}-sensitive Cl conductance of the oocyte to niflumic acid, NFA.[9,10] In the presence of 100 μM NFA, the expressed current was unaffected, whereas the endogenous current was blocked. We also adopted a method first used by Perez to incorporate membrane vesicles derived from cRNA expressing oocytes in to the lipid bilayer.[11] When we did this with oocytes expressing the bovine CLCA and in the presence of niflumic acid, we observed an approximately 21 pS, anion-selective (9:1) and I>Cl (3:1) selective channel. This conductance was activated by Ca^{2+}, and could be blocked by DTT and DIDS. These results were consistent with those that we had previously obtained using the immunopurified protein. However, there was one major discrepancy; whereas the immunopurified protein seemed to consist of multimers of the 38 kDa subunit, the cDNA coded for a protein of

903 amino acids with a predicted molecular mass of approximately 100 kDa. Furthermore, this protein was not susceptible to reduction, despite our observation that DTT could effectively block the expressed conductance. One explanation for this discrepancy is, of course, that the cloned and immunopurified proteins are not in any way related. However, given their functional similarities, we thought this was unlikely, and therefore suggested that the protein derived from the cRNA was subject to post-translational cleavage. This could account for the apparent differences in molecular size and was also feasible as several consensus sites for dibasic proteolytic cleavage were present in the primary amino acid sequence.

2.   THE CLCA FAMILY

Since the cloning of the bovine tracheal CaCC, currently known as bCLCA1, several members of what is an intriguing protein family have been identified. To date, four human and five murine isoforms are known (see Table 1), and there have been examples identified from several other species including rat, pig, and dog.[12-14] However, there are no identified homologs found in C. elegans, Drosophila, yeast or avians. In general the proteins are approximately 900 amino acids long, are predicted to contain both a signal sequence and transmembrane domains, and are indeed post-translationally cleaved into fragments of approximately 100 kDa and 32-38 kDa. The reason why we did not observe the 100 kDa fragment in our immunopurified preparation is most likely because the antibody was raised against the 38 kDa fragment; thus we would have purified the full-length (i.e., pre-cleavage) and 38 kDa polypeptides only. Cleavage seems to be conserved in all family members. The exact number of transmembrane domains present seems to vary dependent on the computer program used for the analysis; however hCLCA2, the only isoform to date to be topology mapped by glycosylation scanning, is predicted to contain five transmembrane domains of which the two most distal are separated in the proteolytic cleavage step.[15] One exception to the predicted membrane location of these proteins is hCLCA3, which has a truncated sequence (262 amino acids) and is secreted when heterologously expressed.[16] The native expression of this protein is extremely low and has led to the suggestion that it may in fact be the product of a pseudogene.[16] It should also be noted that other computer models predict a single transmembrane domain close to the C-terminus.[17,18] Other characteristics of this family include a string of conserved cysteine residues at the N-terminus that conforms to a C-X$_{12}$-C-X$_4$-C-X$_4$-C-X$_{12}$-C repeat. These residues have been postulated to play a role in intermolecular disulfide bonding and may lend some potential structural basis to the inhibition of the channel by the reducing agent DTT.[19] One similarly consistent finding is that all human and mouse CLCAs contain multiple sites for phosphorylation by PKC. The presence of consensus sites for CaMK II and PKA is much more variable (see Tab. 2). However, the presence of a consensus site for kinase phsophorylation does not necessarily translate into a regulatory role for that enzyme, e.g., the bovine CLCA1 was not sensitive to PKA, despite the prediction of consensus phosphorylation sites for this kinase.[9] Members of the family seem to be widely expressed, one isoform or another being found in most tissues and cells, including brain, although an individual family member may exhibit a very restricted pattern of expression; e.g., as determined by Northern blot, hCLCA2 is only expressed to a significant level in trachea and breast tissue, although expression in lung can be detected by RT-PCR.[15]

Table 1. Genbank accession numbers and references of human and murine members of the CLCA family of proteins. mCLCA1 and 2 may represent alternately spliced forms of the same gene. 101 In addition two further mCLCA genes at the same locus as the other murine family members have been identified by data mining. 101 Addition of the rat genome to the NCBI database has revealed three CLCA homologs to date: AB119249, XM217690 and XM342354. The accession number for the porcine variant is AF095584. N.B. The nomenclature is not currently consistent between family members, which were named in the order of which they were cloned. For example, the murine ortholog of hCLCA1 is mCLCA3.

Isoform	GenBank Accession #	Reference
hCLCA1	NM 001285	23, 102
hCLCA2	NM 006536	15, 102, 103
hCLCA3	NM 004921	16
hCLCA4	NM 012128	102
mCLCA1	NM 009899	18, 24
mCLCA2	NM 030601	104
mCLCA3	NM 017474	77
mCLCA4	NM 139148	26
mCLCA5	AY 161007	Elble et al. (unpubl.)

One additional consistent finding in the CLCA family is the presence of a von Willebrand A (VWA) domain. This protein motif is implicated in cell:cell and cell:matrix adhesion in numerous situations and has been found in over 2000 proteins to date.[17] A VWA domain is also found in the $\alpha 2\delta$ subunit of the voltage-sensitive Ca^{2+} channel. This subunit, which is the product of a single gene, consists of two polypeptide cleavage products of a single precursor. The larger cleaved $\alpha 2$ fragment is extracellular and associates via disulfide bonding with the smaller δ fragment which is anchored to the membrane. The heteromeric $\alpha 2\delta$ subunit is thought to interact with the conductive $\alpha 1$ subunit, and regulates trafficking of $\alpha 1$ to the membrane, influences the kinetics of the channel and the current amplitude.[20,21] While some of these features are reminiscent of the situation with the CLCAs, there are some differences. Whereas the 38 kDa fragment (the δ subunit equivalent) may remain associated with the larger 100 kDa polypeptide in the case of hCLCA1, co-precipitation studies suggest that this is not the case for either bCLCA2/Lu-ECAM-1 or hCLCA2.[22,23] In addition, the results of glycosylation scanning combined with a protease protection assay to identify extracellular glycosylated asparagine residues in hCLCA2 was consistent with the presence of multiple transmembrane domains.[15] Furthermore, only transfection in HEK 293 cells of a DNA construct encoding the larger N-terminal portion of hCLCA2 (hCLCA2 R675X) was associated with an increase in thapsigargin-sensitive Cl⁻ current. Transfection of the DNA corresponding to the 38 kDa fragment (hCLCA2 Δ2-674, the fragment within which the transmembrane domain would sit in the single TM model) resulted in no observable current, whereas simultaneous transfection of both plasmids resulted in no more current than that seen for the transfection of the R675X construct alone (Fuller et al. unpublished observations). Thus the role of the VWA domain in the CLCAs remains unclear, as does the role of any association between the larger and smaller cleaved CLCA products at the membrane.

3.   ELECTROPHYSIOLOGY OF THE CLCAS

As described above, the first CLCA family member was cloned from bovine trachea in the mid-1990s.[9] Since then, several homologous polypeptides have been identified in a variety of mammalian species, by a number of different laboratories. Of these, several have been expressed in a variety of heterologous systems and been subjected to eletrophysiological recording. When hCLCA1, hCLCA2 or mCLCA1 were expressed in HEK 293 cells, transfected cells expressed a novel Ca^{2+}-sensitive Cl⁻ current that was not observed in untransfected, mock-transfected or reporter (GFP) transfected cells.[15,23,24] This current could be variably inhibited by a wide range of compounds commonly used as Cl⁻ channel blockers, including niflumic acid (NFA), NPPB and DIDS, although it should be noted that none of these agents are very specific for the CLCAs or any other Cl⁻ channel. Under whole-cell recording conditions with 2 mM Ca^{2+} in the bath and EGTA in the pipette, (free $[Ca^{2+}]_i$ was approximately 100 nM), an outwardly-rectified current of approximately 200 pA average magnitude, could be activated in response to 2 μM ionomycin, a Ca^{2+} ionophore. This current could be blocked by DIDS, niflumic acid and NPPB among others. It was also blocked by addition of DTT to the bath, which we had previously found for the immunopurified protein[7] and which is consistent with inhibition of a multimeric protein. Others have found similar results.[25-27]

Table 2. Number of consensus sites for phosphorylation by PKA, PKC, and CaMK II found in human and murine CLCA family members. Protein sequences were scanned using Scansite software (www.scansite.mit.edu)[105] at medium stringency. The occurrence of C-terminal PDZ domains is also shown.

Isoform	PKA	PKC	CaMK II	PDZ
hCLCA1	1	8	0	1
hCLCA2	0	2	1	0
hCLCA3	2	1	2	0
hCLCA4	0	5	0	1
mCLCA1	4	5	0	0
mCLCA2	4	6	1	0
mCLCA3	0	4	0	0
mCLCA4	1	3	2	0
mCLCA5	1	5	1	1

The currents were time-independent, in contrast to native CaCCs that generally exhibit time-dependent kinetics. The explanation for this difference could be that the HEK cell lacks other components that are required to confer the property of time-dependence on the conductance. Some experimental evidence for this point of view has been reported by Greenwood and colleagues who used HEK 293 cells to co-express the regulatory β subunit of the Ca^{2+}-regulated maxi-K^+ channel with mCLCA1. This maneuver resulted in a whole-cell conductance that was markedly more sensitive to Ca^{2+} than was mCLCA1 alone, and that showed a marked time-dependent activation, very reminiscent of the native CaCC conductance.[28] Subsequent two-hybrid analysis demonstrated that these two proteins might interact in an in vitro system, although whether or not this occurs in vivo needs to be established by co-immunoprecipitation assays. However, this result does raise the intriguing possibility that a CLCA subunit capable of forming heteromeric attachments with multiple partners could impart plasticity on the types of Ca^{2+}-activated Cl^- conductance and/or channel that are recorded in different cells or even within the same cell. Precedence for this is found within the Deg/ENaC family where it is emerging that multiple

ENaC/ASIC channel subunits are co- expressed within a single cell, and may contribute to a multimeric conductance protein.[29] In this regard it is interesting to note that some of the CLCA proteins encode well-conserved PDZ motifs at their C-termini (Table 2).

As noted above, the immunopurified bovine tracheal protein was sensitive to increasing [Ca^{2+}], but its' sensitivity was further increased in the presence of CaMK II. The dose-response curve exhibited a maximum channel open probability at 1 µM [Ca^{2+}].[8] We observed a very similar dose-response relationship for the cloned bCLCA1 protein, the only difference being that the basal open probability of the cloned protein was approximately 0.4.[30] In an attempt to further investigate the Ca^{2+}-dependence of the response, we examined the effect of the inositol polyphosphate, inositol 3,4,5,6-tetrakisphosphate (IP_4) on the cloned bCLCA1 incorporated into planar lipid bilayers. This compound, which is a by-product of the phospholipase C signalling cascade, had been previously shown to inhibit Ca^{2+}-dependent Cl⁻ secretion from T-84 cell monolayers (a colonic carcinoma cell line) under short circuit conditions.[31] Addition of low concentrations of IP_4 (20 nM) caused a leftward shift in the dose-response curve for Ca^{2+} in the absence on CaMK II.[30] Under these conditions, the peak increase in channel P_o occurred at approximately 250 nM [Ca^{2+}], although the maximum P_o only increased to about 0.6. In the presence of CaMK II (+ ATP and calmodulin), peak channel P_o was shifted even further to the left, such that peak opening of approximately 0.9 occurred at a free [Ca^{2+}] of approximately 35 nM. As [Ca^{2+}] was increased above these levels, the channel began to shut down; in the presence of IP_4 and CaMK II, the channel had a P_o of 0.1 at 1 µM [Ca^{2+}]. The distinct biphasic nature of the dose-response curve was exactly what we had seen previously on incorporation of the immunopurified protein into the bilayer and thus was not a consequence of exposure to IP_4.[8] The concentrations of IP_4 used in this study were also significantly lower than the reported intracellular concentrations of IP_4.[32] The implication of this study is that the CLCA protein might not be a very efficient Cl⁻ conductor under conditions of physiological activation of the PLC cascade. IP_4 has been previously shown to be a very effective blocker of the native CaCC in a variety of epithelial cell types.[31, 33-36] However, it should be remembered that the planar lipid bilayer is an artificial system and that accessory proteins that modulate the conductance may not be present. In addition to CaMK II, we have also shown that the bovine CLCA1 protein can be regulated by PKC when expressed in Xenopus oocytes. In the presence of 100 µM niflumic acid to inhibit the endogenous oocyte CaCC, we found that both the wild type and a truncated bCLCA1 were associated with a phorbol ester-sensitive current.[37] This current was completely inhibited by 10 µM chelerythrine chloride, at which concentration it is a specific PKC inhibitor. Interestingly, the current generated by the truncated construct was indistinguishable from the wild-type current, although translation of the mutant initiated at M277 and terminated at R667 retaining the four predicted hydrophobic domains. These observations are consistent with the number of consensus phosphorylation sites for both CaMK II and PKC that are present in the primary amino acid sequence. It should also be noted that one porcine CLCA family member has been reported to be sensitive to phosphorylation by PKA.[38] Heterologous expression in the colonic carcinoma cell line Caco-2 resulted in an increase in cAMP-sensitive Cl⁻ transport.[38] Caco-2 cells do express a small endogenous Ca^{2+}-activated Cl⁻ conductance, which could be augmented by expression of pCLCA1. However, when Caco-2 cells heterologously expressing pCLCA1 were allowed to differentiate, the Ca^{2+}-sensitive Cl⁻ conductance (presumably comprised of both the endogenous and expressed components), was lost, as has been reported for differentiation of many epithelial cells.[39,40] However, the cAMP sensitivity of the Cl⁻ response was retained. This observation has been taken as evidence for pCLCA1 acting as a regulator of the endogenous Ca^{2+}-sensitive Cl⁻ channel, although an alternate possibility is that other proteins required for expression of the conductance are also down-regulated.

A limited number of single channel patch-clamp studies have been carried out with hCLCA1 and bCLCA1.[23,41] When expressed in HEK 293 cells, bCLCA1 had a conductance of approximately 30 pS in the inside-out recording configuration. However, the open probability of the channel was relatively low (0.34 at + 60 mV) at 800 nM free Ca^{2+}. Under cell-attached recording conditions, hCLCA1 exhibited a lower conductance of approximately 13 pS; total current flowing through the patch increased five-fold on exposure of the cell to 2 μM ionomycin.[23]

4.   CLCAS IN CANCER: CELL ADHESION, METASTASIS AND TUMOR SUPPRESSION

The second CLCA homolog identified was bCLCA2, the second bovine isoform. The cloning of this protein was interesting as it was originally isolated as a lung endothelial cell adhesion molecule (Lu-ECAM) by Pauli and collaborators and only identified as a CLCA family member on the basis of sequence analysis that revealed it was 92% identical to bCLCA1.[42] Using specific antibodies, Elble et al. were able to demonstrate that bCLCA2 was indeed subject to post-translational processing that cut the protein into fragments of approximately 90 kDa and 32-38 kDa. A similar pattern of processing has since been found for all other CLCA homologs where it has been examined. The role of bCLCA2 as a cell adhesion molecule is intriguing, but it is by no means unique among the CLCAs in this respect. Monoclonal antibodies directed against bCLCA2 prevented adherence of B16-F10 metastatic melanoma cells to an underlying BAEC substrate expressing bCLCA2/Lu-ECAM I.[43,44] The human isoform hCLCA2, and the murine isoform mCLCA1, also seem to mediate adhesion, specifically interacting with β_4 integrin.[45-47]

A considerable number of studies from the Cornell group have demonstrated the important consequences of CLCA expression or lack thereof for cell adhesion and tumor metastasis. The CLCAs so far examined (mCLCA1 and 2, hCLCA2) play different roles dependent on where they are expressed. When expressed in the tumor cell, the CLCAs appear to act as tumor suppressors. When innoculated into nude mice, metastatic breast cancer cells form fewer and smaller tumors when transfected with hCLCA2 than when transduced with vector alone.[48] Similar results have been observed for mCLCA1 and 2 and it has been suggested that expression of the CLCAs sensitize tumor cells to apoptosis.[49] Importantly, expression of mCLCA1, mCLCA2 and hCLCA2 was significantly down-regulated in highly metastatic breast cancer cell lines.[48,49] This association of CLCA down-regulation with increased metastatic potential may also apply to other cancers; expression of hCLCA1 and 2 was reduced by more than 90% in colonic tumors as compared to paired samples of normal colon. [50] Whereas expression of the CLCAs in the tumor cell may be interpreted as a good thing, expression of the CLCAs in the vascular endothelium is bad if a metastatic tumor is present. Adhesion of the tumor cell to an appropriate substrate is fundamental to the process of metastasis. It has been recently shown that β_4 integrin, which is highly expressed in metastatic melanoma and breast cancer cells is a specific ligand for endothelial CLCAs (mCLCA1, mCLCA5, hCLCA2 and bCLCA2).[47] Non-endothelial CLCAs such as hCLCA1 do not bind β_4 integrin. The endothelial CLCA isoforms thus provide a site of attachment for metastatic tumor cells, which can then initiate colony formation. Attachment to the endothelium is swiftly followed by activation of focal adhesion kinase (FAK) and initiation of the ERK/MAP kinase cascade.[46] This signaling cascade provides the impetus for growth and proliferation of the tumor. Both cleavage products of hCLCA2 contain a functional β_4 integrin binding motif, although in the case of the 35kDa fragment, this domain would be intracellular according to the predicted five transmembrane domain structure for this protein.[15,47] In contrast, the β_4 integrin binding motif in the 90 kDa fragment is located in the second extracellular loop. Importantly, this motif is not conserved in a non-endothelial CLCA, hCLCA1.[47] However, although the binding of β_4 integrin to the CLCAs is required to trigger colony formation, it cannot be wholly sufficient as benign breast tumor cell lines also express this integrin. [45, 46] It is likely that the coordinate expression of several cell surface proteins is necessary for the establishment of metastatic foci.

5. CLCAS IN AIRWAY DISEASE: CYSTIC FIBROSIS AND ASTHMA

Although it had been known from the early work of Quinton and collaborators that the primary defect in cystic fibrosis (CF) was located at the level of a Cl⁻ conductance,[51,52] it was something of a surprise when the defect was found to reside in a member of the ABC family of transport proteins. [53] To date, CFTR is the only member of this family that has been unequivocally shown to be a Cl⁻ channel. The deleterious consequences of a non-expressed or poorly functional CFTR channel for the CF patient are clear; sticky dehydrated secretions in the airways, persistent pulmonary bacterial infections, chronic airway inflammation, and ultimately, for the most severely affected patients, a life expectancy in the low to mid thirties.

However, CFTR is not the only Cl⁻ conductance expressed in the airway epithelial cell. One of the more intriguing paradoxes surrounding CF research is why patients ever get sick from CF at all, given the multiplicity of Cl⁻ current footprints that seem to be expressed in epithelial cells; it would seem as if one of the other non-CFTR Cl⁻ currents could substitute for a mutant CFTR. Notably, both an outwardly-rectified Cl⁻ channel (ORCC) that is activated by PKA-dependent phosphorylation, and a Ca^{2+}-activated Cl⁻ current (CaCC) pathway are expressed in CF cells. In addition, members of the ClC family of Cl⁻ channels, which may or may not include volume-sensitive Cl⁻ conductances have been identified in epithelia of relevance for CF. Some of the discrepancies can be accounted for by invoking the potential role of CFTR as a regulator of other ion channels. This feature of CFTRs' action has been best established for the ORCC, but remains controversial for some other potential CFTR-regulated channels such as ENaC and ROM K.[54-57] However, Ca^{2+}-dependent Cl⁻ channel activity is preserved in human cells of CF origin. In fact there may be a functionally reciprocal relationship between expression of the CaCC and CFTR at least in some tissues;[58-60] why then does the CaCC not substitute for mutant CFTR? In some instances this may in fact be the case; the noted difficulties in making accurate phenotype/genotype correlations in CF further suggest that genetic and/or environmental factors modify the severity of the disease. One illustration of this is found in "long-living" CF mice, which do not express the frank lung pathology associated with CF in man, but in fact succumb to intestinal obstruction.[61-63] It has been suggested that a genetic modifier is responsible for this observation, more precisely that up-regulation of the Ca^{2+}-dependent Cl^- conductance rescues these animals from the pulmonary consequences of CF.[61,62,64,65] Mice bred on a congenic background exhibit a pulmonary pathology much more reminiscent of the human disease profile, and do not exhibit up-regulation of a CaCC.[66]

Is the CaCC of CF tissues synonymous with (a) member(s) of the CLCA family? The CLCAs are certainly expressed in normal and CF airway and CF pancreatic cell lines (HBE, BEAS2B, IB3, CFPAC-1) raised on impermeable supports, and these cell lines show distinctive CaCC currents.[36] Furthermore, Ca^{2+}-sensitive Cl^- currents in airway cells can be effectively inhibited by IP_4.[36] In addition, it has been reported that mCLCA3 is specifically up-regulated in the airway of long-living CF mice.[67] However, the evidence that the CaCC of CF epithelia and the CLCAs are one and the same is largely circumstantial, and in the absence of a CLCA specific blocker, it is difficult to assess with any certainty what the exact contribution of CLCA expression may be to the CaCC. Members of the CLCA family cannot underlie every CaCC; in several instances cells that have robust CaCCs do not express a CLCA isoform.[68,69] It has also been reported that CLCAs are not expressed in murine tracheal epithelial cells from CF mice, despite expression of a Ca^{2+}-activated Cl^- current.[60] Other molecular candidates for the CaCC of CF cells include members of the ClC family and the newly identified bestrophins, although like the CLCAs, neither of these polypeptide families faithfully recapitulate all the characteristics (time-dependence of current activation, expression pattern, activation by Ca^{2+}), associated with the native conductance.[3,4,70]

A second airway disease with which the CLCAs have been associated is asthma. Earlier studies suggested a link between Ca^{2+}-mediated Cl^- secretion and the airway hyper-responsiveness (AHR) associated with asthma. Furthermore, agents that reduce bronchoconstriction, e.g. cromoglycates also seemed to block chloride transport.[71] In the majority of asthma patients, the triggering of AHR includes an allergic component, and a strong link has been established between the $T_{H}2$ (T helper type 2) cytokines IL-9 and IL-13, goblet cell hyperplasia and the induction of mucus production.[72-76] Importantly, expression of a murine member of the CLCA family, mCLCA3 (also known as gob-5 and it's human homolog, hCLCA1,[77] have been linked to the goblet cell hyperplasia and increased mucin production that characterizes the asthmatic airway in both humans and in mouse models of the disease. In ovalbumin-sensitized mice, (a widely used model for allergic asthma), pulmonary expression of mCLCA3 was up-regulated; in contrast, functional knockout of mCLCA3 with an antisense adenoviral construct reduced AHR and mucus production.[78] Similarly, hCLCA1 expression is up-regulated in bronchial goblet cells of asthmatic patients while over-expression of hCLCA1 in a mucoepidermoid cell line was associated with the increased secretion of MUC5AC, one of the major components of respiratory mucus.[79,80] A link between T_H2 cytokines, mCLCA3/hCLCA1 and asthma has also been described. Message for hCLCA1, expression of receptors for IL-9 and mucus production are all increased in asthmatic subjects as compared to healthy controls.[79] In IL-9 transgenic mice, mCLCA3 is specifically induced.[75] A second T_H2 cytokine, IL-13, has also been implicated in mucus over-production in asthma.[72] IL-13 and IL-9 have a complex relationship, although in general, the two cytokines induce many of the same effects. IL-13 can be up-regulated by IL-9, although IL-13 is not required for mucus induction by IL-9.[81] In contrast, in IL-9 knockout mice sensitized with ovalbumin, neither IL-13 production nor airway mucus production were impaired.[82] In addition to its' effects on mucus production, IL-13 induces expression of an apical Ca^{2+}-sensitive Cl conductance in human bronchial epithelial cells.[83,84] Whether or not this IL-13-induced conductance is due to expression of hCLCA1 remains to be determined; however, it has been proposed that channels present on the surface of exocytotic granules, (which may be required for the condensation of granule contents), would become contiguous with the plasma cell membrane on granule fusion.[85] In this context, the localization of mCLCA3 on the membrane of mucus granules in mouse respiratory tissues is highly significant.[86] Interestingly, it has recently been reported that expression of IL-9, IL-9 receptors and hCLCA1 are all increased in the airway of CF patients.[87]

6.   SUMMARY

The CLCA family comprises a highly interesting group of proteins that have potentially very diverse functions within the cell. The physiological role of these proteins is yet to be established. They may be independent ion channels or regulatory subunits of such channels; the data obtained to date would be consistent with either interpretation. Results from lipid bilayer analysis using immunopurified protein are reasonably compelling, but because this is such a sensitive assay, the data could also be interpreted to mean that an otherwise undetectable but tightly bound channel remained associated with the purified protein when it was incorporated into the bilayer. Similarly, electrophysiological data obtained using the cloned CLCAs could suggest that the CLCAs either confer a novel Ca^{2+} sensitivity to a channel or activate an otherwise cryptic conductance. Expression of the bestrophin proteins is associated with the novel appearance of a linear Ca^{2+}- and DIDS-sensitive current in HEK 293 cells.[2-4] However, as shown by

Greenwood and colleagues, co-expression of a CLCA with the BK channel β subunit resulted in a time-dependent conductance with an enhanced sensitivity for Ca^{2+}.[28] One exciting possibility therefore is that the CLCAs may interact with the bestrophins or other proteins to generate the classical CaCC current profile. There may be more to this story: both the CLCAs and the bestrophins are reported to be expressed in the colon,[23,88] despite several reports that Ca^{2+}-activated Cl⁻ secretion does not occur in the gut.[89,90] However, a residual Ca^{2+}-activated Cl⁻ current is found in some severely affected CF patients and in some intestinal cell models.[91-94]

What about the potential role of the CLCAs in cancer? There is certainly precedence in the literature for ion channel subunits to act as cell adhesion molecules,[95-97] and for the involvement of ion channels in cancer progression,[29,98,99] although in this latter role, channels are thought to aid rather than hinder the extreme changes in shape and volume that need to occur during invasion and proliferation. Why channels should be required for apoptosis is currently unknown, although it has been suggested that as the maintenance of a K^+ gradient across the membrane is essential for cellular survival, K^+ efflux may be a "disaster signal" that can trigger apoptosis.[100] In this context, Cl⁻ efflux would be required to maintain electroneutrality. As an increase in cell Ca^{2+} frequently precedes apoptosis, the commonality of Ca^{2+} signaling between these two ion transport pathways is intriguing. Whether the CLCAs need to act as ion channels/regulators in order to be tumor suppressors, or whether these two potential functions are totally independent of one another remains to be determined. Similarly, the reason underlying the seemingly specific up-regulation of CLCA1 in the airways of asthmatic patients and murine models of AHR is unclear; it may be required to promote mucus secretion as part of the inflammatory response of the airway, and perhaps serves a similar role in CF patients. In this case, it might be deleterious to increase expression of CLCA1 in the CF airway. In contrast, the mouse homolog of CLCA1 may act as a positive genetic modifier in long-living CF mice. These apparently contradictory data may suggest that up-regulation of the CLCA in mice may not necessarily translate to the human disease.[101] Clearly the role of this protein in the airway as elsewhere, is an important issue that needs to be resolved.

ACKNOWLEDGEMENTS

Work in the authors' laboratory is supported by NIH Grant DK53090.

REFERENCES

1. P. Huang, J. Liu, A. Di, N. C. Robinson, M. W. Musch, M. A. Kaetzel, and D. J. Nelson. Regulation of human ClC-3 channels by multifunctional Ca^{2+}/calmodulin-dependent protein kinase. *J. Biol. Chem.* **276**, 20093-20100 (2001).
2. H. Sun, T. Tsunenari, K. W. Yau, and J. Nathans. The vitelliform macular dystrophy protein defines a new family of chloride channels. *Proc. Natl. Acad. Sci. U. S. A.* **99**, 4008-4013 (2002).
3. T. Tsunenari, H. Sun, J. Williams, H. Cahill, P. Smallwood, K. W. Yau, and J. Nathans. Structure-function analysis of the bestrophin family of anion channels. *J. Biol. Chem.* **278**, 41114-41125 (2003).
4. Z. Qu, R. W. Wei, W. Mann and H. C. Hartzell. Two bestrophins cloned from Xenopus laevis oocytes express Ca^{2+}-activated Cl⁻ currents. *J. Biol. Chem.* **278**, 49563-49572 (2003).
5. S. Ran and D. J. Benos. Isolation and functional reconstitution of a 38-kDa chloride channel protein from bovine tracheal membranes. *J. Biol. Chem.* **266**, 4782-4788 (1991).
6. S. Rana and D. J. Benos. Immunopurification and structural analysis of a putative epithelal Cl⁻ channel protein isolated from bovine trachea. *J. Biol. Chem.* **267**, 3618-3625 (1992).
7. S. Ran, C. M. Fuller, M. P. Arrate, R. Latorre and D. J. Benos. Functional reconstitution of a chloride channel protein from bovine trachea. *J. Biol. Chem.* **267**, 20630-20637 (1992).
8. C. M. Fuller, I. I. Ismailov, D. Keeton, and D. J. Benos. Phosphorylation and activation of an anion channel from bovine trachea by Ca^{2+}/calmodulin dependent kinase II. *J. Biol. Chem.* **269**, 26642-26650 (1994).
9. S. A. Cunningham, M. S. Awayda, J. K. Bubien, I. I. Ismailov, M. P. Arrate, B. K. Berdiev, D. J. Benos, and C. M. Fuller. Cloning of an epithelial chloride channel from bovine trachea. *J. Biol. Chem.* **270**, 31016-31026 (1995).
10. M. M. White and M. Aylwin. Niflumic and flufenamic acids are potent reversible blockers of Ca^{2+}-activated Cl⁻ channels in Xenopus oocytes. *Mol. Pharmacol.* **37**, 720-724 (1990).
11. G. Perez, A. Lagrutta, J. P. Adelman, and L. Toro. Reconstitution of expressed KCa channels from Xenopus oocytes to lipid bilayers. *Biophys. J.* **66**, 1022-1027 (1994).
12. F. Thevenod, E. Roussa, D. J. Benos, and C. M. Fuller. Relationship between a HCO_3^--permeable conductance and a CLCA protein from rat pancreatic zymogen granules. *Biochem. Biophys. Res. Commun.* **300**, 546-554 (2003).
13. M. E. Loewen, N. K. Smith, D. L. Hamilton, B. H. Grahn, and G. W. Forsyth. CLCA protein and chloride transport in canine retinal pigment epithelium. *Am. J. Physiol. Cell Physiol.* **285**, C1314-1321 (2003).
14. K. J. Gaspar, K. J. Racette, J. R. Gordon, M. E. Loewen, and G. W. Forsyth. Cloning a chloride conductance mediator from the apical membrane of porcine ileal enterocytes. *Physiol. Genomics* **3**, 101-111 (2000).
15. A. D. Gruber, K. D. Schreur, H.-L. Ji, C. M. Fuller, and B. U. Pauli. Molecular cloning and transmembrane structure of hCLCA2 from human lung, trachea and mammary gland. *Am. J. Physiol. Cell Physiol.* **276**, C1261-1270 (1999).
16. A. D. Gruber and B. U. Pauli. Molecular cloning and biochemical characterization of a truncated, secreted member of the human family of Ca^{2+}-activated Cl⁻ channels. *Biochim. Biophys. Acta* **1444**, 418-423 (1999).
17. C. A. Whittaker and R. O. Hynes. Distribution and evolution of von Willebrand/integrin A domains: widely dispersed domains with roles in cell adhesion and elsewhere. *Mol. Biol. Cell* **13**, 3369-3387 (2002).

18. L. Romio, L. Musante, R. Cinti, M. Seri, O. Moran, O. Zegarra-Moran, and L. J. Galietta. Characterization of a murine gene homologous to the bovine CaCC chloride channel. *Gene* **228**, 181-188 (1999).
19. A. D. Gruber, C. M. Fuller, R. C. Elble, D. J. Benos, and B. U. Pauli. The CLCA gene family: a novel family of putative chloride channels. *Curr. Genomics* **1**, 201-222 (2000).
20. M. Hobom, S. Dai, E. Marais, L. Lacinova, F. Hofmann, and N. Klugbauer. Neuronal distribution and functional characterization of the calcium channel alpha2delta-2 subunit. *Eur. J. Neurosci.* **12**, 1217-1226 (2000).
21. J. Arikkath and K. P. Campbell. Auxiliary subunits: essential components of the voltage-gated calcium channel complex. *Curr. Opin. Neurobiol.* **13**, 298-307 (2003).
22. A. D. Gruber, R. C. Elble, and B.U. Pauli. Discovery and cloning of the CLCA gene family. In: *Calcium-activated Chloride Channels*. Edited by C.M. Fuller (Elsevier/Academic Press, San Diego, 2002), Vol. **53**, pp. 367-387.
23. A. D. Gruber, R. C. Elble, H.-L. Ji, K. D. Schreur, C. M. Fuller, and B. U. Pauli. Genomic cloning, molecular characterization, and functional analysis of human CLCA1, the first human member of the family of Ca^{2+}-activated Cl⁻ channel proteins. *Genomics* **54**, 200-214 (1998).
24. R. Gandhi, R. C. Elble, A. D. Gruber, K. D. Schreur, H.-L. Ji, C. M. Fuller, and B. U. Pauli. Molecular and functional characterization of a calcium-sensitive chloride channel from mouse lung. *J. Biol. Chem.* **273**, 32096-32101 (1998).
25. G. S. Stewart, M. Glanville, O. Aziz, N. L. Simmons, and M. A. Gray. Regulation of an outwardly rectifying chloride conductance in renal epithelial cells by external and internal calcium. *J. Membr. Biol.* **180**, 49-64 (2001).
26. R. C. Elble, G. Ji, K. Nehrke, J. DeBiasio, P. D. Kingsley, M. I. Kotlikoff, and B. U. Pauli. Molecular and functional characterization of a murine calcium-activated chloride channel expressed in smooth muscle. *J. Biol. Chem.* **277**, 18586-18591 (2002).
27. F. C. Britton, S. Ohya, B. Horowitz, and I. A. Greenwood. Comparison of the properties of CLCA1 generated currents and I(Cl(Ca)) in murine portal vein smooth muscle cells. *J. Physiol.* **539**, 107-117 (2002).
28. I. A. Greenwood, L. J. Miller, S. Ohya, and B. Horowitz. The large conductance potassium channel beta-subunit can interact with and modulate the functional properties of a calcium-activated chloride channel, CLCA1. *J. Biol. Chem.* **277** 22119-22122 (2002).
29. B. K. Berdiev, J. Xia, L. A. McLean, J. M. Markert, G. Y. Gillespie, T. B. Mapstone, A. P. Naren, B. Jovov, J. K. Bubien, H. L. Ji *et al.* Acid-sensing ion channels in malignant gliomas. *J. Biol. Chem.* **278**, 15023-15034 (2003).
30. I. I. Ismailov, C. M. Fuller, B. K. Berdiev, D. J. Benos, and K. E. Barrett. A biologic function for an "orphan" messenger: D-myo-inositol (3,4,5,6)tetrakisphosphate selectively blocks epithelial calcium-activated chloride channels. *Proc. Natl. Acad. Sci. U.S.A.* **93**, 10505-10509 (1996).
31. M. Vajanaphanich, C. Schultz, M. T. Rudolf, M. Wasserman, P. Enyedi, A. Craxton, S. B. Shears, R. Y. Tsien, K. E. Barrett, and A. E. Traynor-Kaplan. Long-term uncoupling of chloride secretion from intracellular calcium levels by Ins(3,4,5,6)P_4. *Nature* **371**, 711-714 (1994).
32. M. W. Y. Ho and S. B. Shears. Regulation of calcium-activated chloride channels by inositol 3,4,5,6-tetrakisphosphate. In: *Calcium-activated Chloride Channels*. Edited by C.M. Fuller (Elsevier/Academic Press, San Diego, 2002), Vol. **53**, pp. 345-363.
33. M. A. Carew, X. Yang, C. Schultz, and S. B. Shears. myo-Inositol 3,4,5,6-tetrakisphosphate inhibits an apical calcium-activated chloride conductance in polarized monolayers of a cystic fibrosis cell line. *J. Biol. Chem.* **275**, 26906-26913 (2000).

34. M. W. Ho, S. B. Shears, K. S. Bruzik, M. Duszyk, and A. S. French. Ins(3,4,5,6)P_4 inhibits a receptor-mediated Ca^{2+}-dependent Cl^- current in CFPAC-1 cells. *Am. J. Physiol. Cell Physiol.* **272**, C1160-1168 (1997).

35. M. T. Rudolf, C. Dinkel, A. E. Traynor-Kaplan, and C. Schultz. Antagonists of myoinositol 3,4,5,6-tetrakisphosphate allow repeated epithelial chloride secretion. *Bioorg. Med. Chem.* **11**, 3315-3329 (2003).

36. H. Zhang, S. Parker, K. E. Barrett, D. J. Benos, and C. M. Fuller. Ca^{2+}-activated Cl^- conductances in cultured airway epithelia. *FASEB J.*, **15**, A847 (2001).

37. H.-L. Ji, M. D. DuVall, H. K. Patton, C. L. Satterfield, C. M. Fuller, and D. J. Benos. Functional expression of a truncated epithelial Cl^- channel and activation by phorbol ester. *Am. J. Physiol. Cell Physiol.* **274**, C455-464 (1998).

38. M. E. Loewen, L. K. Bekar, S. E. Gabriel, W. Walz, and G. W. Forsyth. pCLCA1 becomes a cAMP-dependent chloride conductance mediator in Caco-2 cells. *Biochem. Biophys. Res. Commun.* **298**, 531-536 (2002).

39. M. E. Loewen, L. K. Bekar, W. Walz, G. W. Forsyth, and S. E. Gabriel. pCLCA1 lacks inherent chloride channel activity in an epithelial colon carcinoma cell line. *Am. J. Physiol. Gastrointest. Liver Physiol.* in press (2004).

40. M. P. Anderson and M. J. Welsh. Calcium and cAMP activate different chloride channels in the apical membrane of normal and cystic fibrosis epithelia. *Proc. Natl. Acad. Sci. U.S.A.* **88**, 6003-6007 (1991).

41. C. M. Fuller and D. J. Benos. Electrophysiology of the CLCA family. In: *Calcium-activated Chloride Channels.* Edited by C.M. Fuller (Elsevier/Academic Press, San Diego, 2002), Vol. **53**, pp. 389-414.

42. R. C. Elble, J. Widom, A. D. Gruber, M. Abdel-Ghany, R. Levine, A. Goodwin, H.-C. Cheng, B. U. Pauli. Cloning and characterization of lung-endothelial cell adhesion molecule-1 suggest it is an endothelial chloride channel. *J. Biol. Chem.* **272**, 27853-27861 (1997).

43. D. Z. Zhu, C. F. Cheng, and B. U. Pauli. Mediation of lung metastasis of murine melanomas by a lung-specific endothelial cell adhesion molecule. *Proc. Natl. Acad. Sci. U. S. A.* **88**, 9568-9572 (1991).

44. D. Zhu, C. F. Cheng, and B. U. Pauli. Blocking of lung endothelial cell adhesion molecule-1 (Lu-ECAM-1) inhibits murine melanoma lung metastasis. *J. Clin. Invest.* **89**, 1718-1724 (1992).

45. M. Abdel-Ghany, H.-C. Cheng, R. C. Elble, and B. U. Pauli. The breast cancer β_4 integrin and endothelial human CLCA2 mediate lung metastasis. *J. Biol. Chem.* **276**, 25438-25446 (2001).

46. M. Abdel-Ghany, H. C. Cheng, R. C. Elble, and B. U. Pauli. Focal adhesion kinase activated by beta(4) integrin ligation to mCLCA1 mediates early metastatic growth. *J. Biol. Chem.* **277**, 34391-34400 (2002).

47. M. Abdel-Ghany, H. C. Cheng, R. C. Elble, H. Lin, J. DiBiasio, and B. U. Pauli. The Interacting Binding Domains of the {beta}4 Integrin and Calcium-activated Chloride Channels (CLCAs) in Metastasis. *J. Biol. Chem.* **278**, 49406-49416 (2003).

48. A. D. Gruber and B. U. Pauli. Tumorigenicity of human breast cancer is associated with loss of the Ca^{2+}-activated chloride channel CLCA2. *Cancer Res.* **59**, 5488-5491 (1999).

49. R. C. Elble and B. U. Pauli. Tumor suppression by a proapoptotic calcium-activated chloride channel in mammary epithelium. *J. Biol. Chem.* **276**, 40510-40517 (2001).

50. S. A. Bustin, S. R. Li, and S. Dorudi. Expression of the Ca^{2+}-activated chloride channel genes CLCA1 and CLCA2 is downregulated in human colorectal cancer. *DNA Cell Biol.* **20**, 331-338 (2001).

51. P. M. Quinton and J. Bijman. Higher bioelectric potentials due to decreased chloride absorption in the sweat glands of patients with cystic fibrosis. *N. Engl. J Med.* **308**, 1185-1189 (1983).
52. P. M. Quinton. Chloride impermeability in cystic fibrosis. *Nature* **301**, 421-422 (1983).
53. J. R. Riordan, J. M. Rommens, B. Kerem, N. Alon, R. Rozmahel, Z. Grzelczak, J. Zielenski, S. Lok, N. Plavsic, J. L. Chou *et al*. Identification of the cystic fibrosis gene: cloning and characterization of complementary DNA. *Science* **245**, 1066-1073 (1989).
54. K. Ho. The ROMK-cystic fibrosis transmembrane conductance regulator connection: new insights into the relationship between ROMK and cystic fibrosis transmembrane conductance regulator channels. *Curr. Opin. Nephrol. Hypertens.* **7**, 49-58 (1998).
55. I. I. Ismailov, M. S. Awayda, B. J. Jovov, B. K. Berdiev, C. M. Fuller, J. R ⌐edman, and D. J. Benos. Regulation of epithelial sodium channels by the cysuc fibrosis transmembrane conductance regulator. *J. Biol. Chem.* **271**, 4725-4732 (1996).
56. K. Kunzelmann. ENaC is inhibited by an increase in the intracellular Cl(-) concentration mediated through activation of Cl(-) channels. *Pflug. Arch.-Eur.J. Physiol.* **445**, 504-512 (2003).
57. M. J. Stutts, C. M. Canessa, J. C. Olsen, M. Hamrick, J. A. Cohn, B. C. Rossier, and R. C. Boucher. CFTR as a cAMP-dependent regulator of sodium channels. *Science* **269**, 847-850 (1995).
58. T. Chinet, L. Fouassier, N. Dray-Charier, M. Imam-Ghali, H. Morel, M. Mergey, B. Dousset, R. Parc, A. Paul, and C. Housset. Regulation of electrogenic anion secretion in normal and cystic fibrosis gallbladder mucosa. *Hepatol.* **29**, 5-13 (1999).
59. L. G. Johnson, S. E. Boyles, J. Wilson, and R. C. Boucher. Normalization of raised sodium absorption and raised calcium-mediated chloride secretion by adenovirus-mediated expression of cystic fibrosis transmembrane conductance regulator in primary human cystic fibrosis airway epithelial cells. *J. Clin. Invest.* **95**, 1377-1382 (1995).
60. R. Tarran, M. E. Loewen, A. M. Paradiso, J. C. Olsen, M. A. Gray, B. E. Argent, R. C. Boucher, and S. E. Gabriel. Regulation of murine airway surface liquid volume by CFTR and Ca^{2+}-activated Cl$^-$ conductances. *J. Gen. Physiol.* **120**, 407-418 (2002).
61. L. L. Clarke, B. R. Grubb, S. E. Gabriel, O. Smithies, B. H. Koller, and R. C. Boucher. Defective epithelial chloride transport in a gene targeted mouse model of cystic fibrosis. *Science* **257**, 1125-1128 (1992).
62. B. R. Grubb, R. N. Vick, and R. C. Boucher. Hyperabsorption of Na$^+$ and raised Ca^{2+}-mediated Cl$^-$ secretion in nasal epithelia of CF mice. *Am. J. Physiol. Cell Physiol.* **266**, C1478-1483 (1994).
63. B. R. Grubb and R. C. Boucher. Pathophysiology of gene-targeted mouse models for cystic fibrosis. *Physiol. Rev.* **79**, S193-214 (1999).
64. C. K. Haston, C. McKerlie, S. Newbigging, M. Corey, R. Rozmahel, and L. C. Tsui: Detection of modifier loci influencing the lung phenotype of cystic fibrosis knockout mice. *Mamm. Genome* **13**, 605-613 (2002).
65. R. Rozmahel, M. Wilschanski, A. Matin, S. Plyte, M. Oliver, W. Auerbach, A. Moore, J. Forstner, P. Durie, J. Nadeau *et al*. Modulation of disease severity in cystic fibrosis transmembrane conductance regulator deficient mice by a secondary genetic factor. *Nature Genet.* **12**, 280-287 (1996).
66. G. Kent, R. Iles, C. E. Bear, L.-J. Huan, U. Griesenbach, C. McKerlie, H. Frndova, C. Ackerley, D. Gosselin, D. Radzioch *et al*. Lung disease in mice with cystic fibrosis. *J. Clin. Invest.* **100**, 3060-3069 (1997).
67. C. Chung, I. Fang, V. Nguyen, C. KLuk, G. Kent, and R. Rozmahel. Investigation of mCLCA3 as a modifier of CF disease in mice. *Ped. Pulm.* **22** Suppl., 217 (2001).

68. P. Fong, B. E. Argent, W. B. Guggino, and M. A. Gray. Characterization of vectorial chloride transport pathways in the human pancreatic duct adenocarcinoma cell line HPAF. *Am. J. Physiol. Cell Physiol.* **285**, C433-445 (2003).

69. J. Papassotiriou, J. Eggermont, G. Droogmans, and B. Nilius. Ca^{2+}-activated Cl⁻ channels in Ehrlich ascites tumor cells are distinct from mCLCA1, 2 and 3. *Pflug. Arch.-Eur. J. Physiol.* **442**, 273-279 (2001).

70. C.M. Fuller and D.J. Benos. Ca^{2+}-activated Cl⁻ channels: a newly emerging anion transport family. *News Physiol. Sci.* **15**, 165-171 (2000).

71. E. W. Alton, D. J. Kingsleigh-Smith, F. M. Munkonge, S. N. Smith, A. R. Lindsay, D. C. Gruenert, P. K. Jeffery, A. Norris, D. M. Geddes, and A.J. Williams. Asthma prophylaxis agents alter the function of an airway epithelial chloride channel. *Am. J. Respir. Cell Mol. Biol.* **14**, 380-387 (1996).

72. D. A. Kuperman, X. Huang, L. L. Koth, G. H. Chang, G. M. Dolganov, Z. Zhu, J. A. Elias, D. Sheppard, and D. J. Erle. Direct effects of interleukin-13 on epithelial cells cause airway hyperreactivity and mucus overproduction in asthma. *Nat. Med.* **8**, 885-889 (2002).

73. J. Louahed, M. Toda, J. Jen, Q. Hamid, J. C. Renauld, R. C. Levitt, and N. C. Nicolaides. Interleukin-9 upregulates mucus expression in the airways. *Am. J. Respir. Cell Mol. Biol.* **22**, 649-656 (2000).

74. P. D. Vermeer, R. Harson, L. A. Einwalter, T. Moninger, and J. Zabner. Interleukin-9 induces goblet cell hyperplasia during repair of human airway epithelia. *Am. J. Respir. Cell Mol. Biol.* **28**, 286-295 (2003).

75. Y. Zhou, Q. Dong, J. Louahed, C. Dragwa, D. Savio, M. Huang, C. Weiss, Y. Tomer, M. P. McLane, N. C. Nicolaides *et al.* Characterization of a calcium-activated chloride channel as a shared target of Th2 cytokine pathways and its potential involvement in asthma. *Am. J. Respir. Cell Mol. Biol.* **25**, 486-491 (2001).

76. Y. Zhou, M. McLane, and R. C. Levitt. Th2 cytokines and asthma. Interleukin-9 as a therapeutic target for asthma. *Respir. Res.* **2**, 80-84 (2001).

77. T. Komiya, Y. Tanigawa, and S. Hirohashi. Cloning and identification of the gene gob-5, which is expressed in intestinal goblet cells in mice. *Biochem. Biophys. Res. Commun.* **255**, 347-351 (1999).

78. A. Nakanishi, S. Morita, H. Iwashita, Y. Sagiya, Y. Ashida, H. Shirafuji, Y. Fujisawa, O. Nishimura, and M. Fujino. Role of gob-5 in mucus overproduction and airway hyperresponsiveness in asthma. *Proc. Natl. Acad. Sci. U.S.A.* **98**, 5175-5180 (2001).

79. M. Toda, M. K. Tulic, R. C. Levitt, and Q. Hamid. A calcium-activated chloride channel (HCLCA1) is strongly related to IL-9 expression and mucus production in bronchial epithelium of patients with asthma. *J. Allergy Clin. Immunol.* **109**, 246-250 (2002).

80. M. Hoshino, S. Morita, H. Iwashita, Y. Sagiya, T. Nagi, A. Nakanishi, Y. Ashida, O. Nishimura, Y. Fujisawa, and M. Fujino. Increased expression of the human Ca^{2+}-activated Cl⁻ channel 1 (CaCC1) gene in the asthmatic airway. *Am. J. Respir. Crit. Care Med.* **165**, 1132-1136 (2002).

81. J.R. Reader, D.M. Hyde, E.S. Schelegle, M.C. Aldrich, A.M. Stoddard, M.P. McLane, R.C. Levitt, J.S. Tepper: Interleukin-9 induces mucous cell metaplasia independent of inflammation. *Am. J. Respir. Cell Mol. Biol.*, **28**,664-672 (2003).

82. S. J. McMillan, B. Bishop, M. J. Townsend, A. N. McKenzie, and C. M. Lloyd. The absence of interleukin 9 does not affect the development of allergen-induced pulmonary inflammation nor airway hyperreactivity. *J. Exp. Med.* **195**, 51-57 (2002).

83. H. Atherton, J. Mesher, C. T. Poll, and H. Danahay. Preliminary pharmacological characterisation of an interleukin-13-enhanced calcium-activated chloride conductance in

the human airway epithelium. *Naunyn Schmiedebergs Arch. Pharmacol.* **367**, 214-217 (2003).

84. H. Danahay, H. Atherton, G. Jones, R. J. Bridges, and C. T. Poll. Interleukin-13 induces a hypersecretory ion transport phenotype in human bronchial epithelial cells. *Am. J. Physiol. Lung Cell Mol. Physiol.* **282**, L226-236 (2002).

85. F. Thevenod. Ion channels in secretory granules of the pancreas and their role in exocytosis and release of secretory proteins. *Am. J Physiol. Cell Physiol.* **283**, C651-672 (2002).

86. I. Leverkoehne and A. D. Gruber. The murine mCLCA3 (alias gob-5) protein is located in the mucin granule membranes of intestinal, respiratory, and uterine goblet cells. *J. Histochem. Cytochem.* **50**, 829-838 (2002).

87. H. P. Hauber, J. J. Manoukian, L. H. Nguyen, S. E. Sobol, R. C. Levitt, K. J. Holroyd, N. G. McElvaney, S. Griffin, and Q. Hamid. Increased expression of interleukin-9, interleukin-9 receptor, and the calcium-activated chloride channel hCLCA1 in the upper airways of patients with cystic fibrosis. *Laryngoscope* **113**, 1037-1042 (2003).

88. H. Stohr, A. Marquardt, I. Nanda, M. Schmid, and B. H. Weber. Three novel human VMD2-like genes are members of the evolutionary highly conserved RFP-TM family. *Eur. J. Hum. Genet.* **10**, 281-284 (2002).

89. H. M. Berschneider, M. R. Knowles, R. G. Azizkhan, R. C. Boucher, N. A. Tobey, R. C. Orlando, and D. W. Powell. Altered intestinal chloride transport in cystic fibrosis. *FASEB J.* **2**, 2625-2629 (1988).

90. J. Hardcastle, P. T. Hardcastle, C. J. Taylor, and J. Goldhill. Failure of cholinergic stimulation to induce a secretory response from the rectal mucosa in cystic fibrosis. *Gut* **32**, 1035-1039 (1991).

91. I. Bronsveld, F. Mekus, J. Bijman, M. Ballmann, J. Greipel, J. Hundrieser, D. J. Halley, U. Laabs, R. Busche, H. R. De Jonge *et al.* Residual chloride secretion in intestinal tissue of deltaF508 homozygous twins and siblings with cystic fibrosis. The European CF Twin and Sibling Study Consortium. *Gastroenterol.* **119**, 32-40 (2000).

92. K.E. Barrett. Calcium-mediated chloride secretion in the intestinal epithelium: significance and regulation. In: *Calcium-activated Chloride Channels.* Edited by C.M. Fuller (Elsevier/Academic Press, San Diego, 2002), Vol. **53**, pp. 257-282.

93. G. T. McEwan, B. H. Hirst, and N. L. Simmons. Carbachol stimulates Cl⁻ secretion via activation of two distinct apical Cl⁻ pathways in cultured human T84 intestinal epithelial monolayers. *Biochim. Biophys. Acta* **1220**, 241-247 (1994).

94. D. Merlin, L. Jiang, G. R. Strohmeier, A. Nusrat, S. L. Alper, W. I. Lencer, and J. L. Madara. Distinct Ca^{2+}- and cAMP-dependent anion conductances in the apical membrane of polarized T84 cells. *Am. J. Physiol. Cell Physiol.* **275**, C484-C495 (1998).

95. J. Liu, B. Schrank, and R.H. Waterston. Interaction between a putative mechanosensory membrane channel and a collagen. *Science* **273**, 361-364 (1996).

96. J. Garcia-Anoveros, J. A. Garcia, J. D. Liu, and D. P. Corey. The nematode degenerin UNC-105 forms ion channels that are activated by degeneration- or hypercontraction-causing mutations. *Neuron* **20**, 1231-1241 (1998).

97. L.L. Isom. The role of sodium channels in cell adhesion. *Front. Biosci.* **7**, 12-23 (2002).

98. S. Roger, P. Besson, and J. Y. Le Guennec. Involvement of a novel fast inward sodium current in the invasion capacity of a breast cancer cell line. *Biochim. Biophys. Acta.* **1616**, 107-111 (2003).

99. H. Sontheimer. Malignant gliomas: perverting glutamate and ion homeostasis for selective advantage. *Trends Neurosci.* **26**, 543-549 (2003).

100. S. P. Yu. Regulation and critical role of potassium homeostasis in apoptosis. *Prog. Neurobiol.* **70**, 363-386 (2003).

101. M. Ritzka, C. Weinel, F. Stanke, and B. Tummler. Sequence comparison of the whole murine and human CLCA locus reveals conserved synteny between both species. *Genome Lett.* **2**,149-154 (2003).

102. M. Agnel, T. Vermat, and J.-M. Culouscou. Identification of three novel members of the calcium-dependent chloride channel (CaCC) family predominantly expressed in the digestive tract and trachea. *FEBS Lett.* **455**, 295-301 (1999).

103. R. Itoh, S. Kawamoto, Y. Miyamoto, S. Kinoshita, and K. Okubo. Isolation and characterization of a Ca^{2+}-activated chloride channel from human corneal epithelium. *Curr. Eye Res.*, **21**,918-925 (2000).

104. D. Lee, S. Ha, Y. Kho, J. Kim, K. Cho, M. Baik, and Y. Choi. Induction of mouse Ca^{2+}-sensitive chloride channel 2 gene during involution of mammary gland. *Biochem. Biophys. Res. Commun.* **264**, 933-937 (1999).

105. M. B. Yaffe, G. G. Leparc, J. Lai, T. Obata, S. Volinia, and L. C. Cantley. A motif-based profile scanning approach for genome-wide prediction of signaling pathways. *Nat. Biotechnol.* **19**, 348-353 (2001).

Chapter 8

IS INTERVENTION IN INOSITOL PHOSPHATE SIGNALING A USEFUL THERAPEUTIC OPTION FOR CYSTIC FIBROSIS?

Stephen B. Shears[1], Ling Yang[1], Sherif Gabriel[2], and Carla M. Pedrosa Ribeiro[2]

[1]*Inositol Signaling Section, Laboratory of Signal Transduction, N.I.E.H.S. / N.I.H. / D.H.S.S., Research Triangle Park, NC 27709, USA, Fax 919-541-0559, Phone 919-541-0793, Email: shears@niehs.nih.gov;* [2]*Department of Pediatrics and Cystic Fibrosis/Pulmonary Research and Treatment Center, University of North Carolina at Chapel Hill, Chapel Hill, NC 27599, USA*

1.   INTRODUCTION

Defects in salt and fluid transport across airway epithelia contribute to the pulmonary manifestation of the cystic fibrosis (CF) condition.[1] Two Cl⁻ conductances have been described in the apical membrane of both human and murine proximal airway epithelia: First, CFTR, which is cAMP-regulated and second, the Ca^{2+}-activated Cl⁻ conductances (CaCC); the molecular identity of the latter channels is uncertain. In humans, the loss of CFTR is a catastrophic event, and currently no drugs with proven safety and efficacy are available to treat this debilitating disease.[2] One of the main areas of study for both genetic and pharmacological treatment of CF is the possibility of up-regulation of the CaCC pathway.[2] One potential means of achieving this goal is activation of CaCC by metabolically-stable, $P2Y_2$ purinergic agonists.[2,3] This in turn could prevent the formation of viscous, dehydrated mucus; periciliary fluid viscosity should improve, fresh mucin secretion would be increased, along with increased ciliary beat frequency.[3] Overall, these activities are predicted to improve airway mucociliary clearance.[3] One potential problem with this approach, that is not widely appreciated, is that prolonged purinergic activation of the inositol signaling pathway leads to the intracellular accumulation of inositol 3,4,5,6-tetrakisphosphate $(Ins(3,4,5,6)P_4)$.[4] The latter is an inhibitor of the very chloride channels that the purinergic agonists are designed to activate.[4-6] This has led to the idea that antagonism of the $Ins(3,4,5,6)P_4$ signaling pathway might be useful as a CF therapy.[7] We will examine these ideas in this review.

2. P2Y$_2$ RECEPTOR-DEPENDENT PHOSPHOLIPASE C (PLC) ACTIVATION AND CA^{2+}-DEPENDENT CHLORIDE SECRETION IN AIRWAY EPITHELIA

The first study demonstrating the coupling between purinoceptor activation and PLC∃ activity in human airway epithelia was performed in the cell line CF/T43 derived from a cystic fibrosis (CF) patient.[8] In that investigation, either extracellular ATP or UTP activated a common 5'-nucleotide or P_{2U}-purinergic (now P2Y$_2$) receptor, which promoted the accumulation of $Ins(1,4,5)P_3$ and other inositol phosphates. This process results in an intracellular Ca^{2+} mobilization through two coupled pathways. Initially, $Ins(1,4,5)P_3$ opens Ca^{2+} channels in the endoplasmic reticulum (ER), resulting in release of stored Ca^{2+} into the cytoplasm. The depletion of ER Ca^{2+} stores subsequently activates a Ca^{2+} influx across the plasma membrane by a process that was originally termed "capacitative Ca^{2+} entry"[9,10] or, more recently, "store-operated calcium entry".[11] Both phases of Ca^{2+} mobilization - release from ER and influx across the plasma membrane - can act together to activate the apical CaCC. Ca^{2+} also has the effect of simultaneously activating Ca^{2+}-dependent K$^+$ channels in the basolateral membrane, thereby providing an electrochemical gradient that favours apical Cl$^-$ exit. Thus, inhibition of basolateral K$^+$ channels inhibits Ca^{2+}-activated Cl$^-$ secretion from airway epithelia.[12]

Sustained transepithelial Cl$^-$ secretion requires more Cl$^-$ to enter the cell through basolateral Na$^+$/K$^+$/2Cl$^-$ cotransporters. Finally, the increased movement of Cl$^-$ across the epithelial monolayer is accompanied by paracellular movement of Na$^+$ and an osmotically driven movement of water.[13,14] The importance of P2Y$_2$ receptors in this entire process has been verified with P2Y$_2$ receptor (-/-) mice in which there is near-complete elimination of nucleotide-stimulated Cl$^-$ secretion from tracheal cells.[15]

3.   REGULATION OF CACC IN NORMAL AND CF AIRWAY EPITHELIA

Airway epithelia are exposed to different mucosal and serosal milieus and they can adapt to these distinct environments by confining physiological functions to their apical or basolateral domains. Activation of either apical or basolateral $P2Y_2$ receptors has been used to demonstrate membrane-specific Ca^{2+}-dependent responses in airway epithelia, since the resulting Ca^{2+} signals triggered by nucleotide exposure can be largely restricted to the membrane domain ipsilateral to receptor activation.[16-18] For example, in monolayers of CF airway epithelia, apical $P2Y_2$ receptor activation-dependent Ca^{2+} mobilization more efficiently couples to apical Cl^- secretion through CaCC than does Ca^{2+} mobilization through basolateral $P2Y_2$ receptor activation.[17,19] On the contrary, Ca^{2+} signals resulting from basolateral $P2Y_2$ receptor activation suffer from considerable attenuation as they traverse through the interior of the epithelial cell to the apical membrane. An important therapeutic point to arise from this idea is that the inhalation of purinergic agonists will serve to activate receptors on the apical surface of the lung epithelia, where they will be especially effective at activating CaCC.

By studying the distribution and the Ca^{2+}-buffering activity of mitochondria in polarized airway epithelia, it has been possible to study the mechanism for the apical membrane-restricted regulation of CaCC. In airway epithelial cells, mitochondria are present at both the apical and the basolateral domains, but they are more concentrated at the apical region and closely associated with the ER.[18] Activation of $P2Y_2$ receptors promoted mitochondrial Ca^{2+} (Ca^{2+}_m) accumulation only in mitochondria localized to the domain ipsilateral to receptor activation, and mitochondrial uncoupling blocked the $P2Y_2$ receptor activation-induced Ca^{2+}_m uptake.[18]

The typical view of Ca^{2+}-activated salt and fluid secretion from polarized epithelia is that activation of basolateral K^+ channels is necessary so as to provide an electrochemical gradient that favours Cl^- exit at the apical pole.[13,14] Indeed, the inhibition of basolateral K^+ channels by clotrimazole can reduce the activity of CaCC in the apical membrane of polarized airway epithelial cells.[12] However, the mitochondrial screen around the apical pole limits the movement of Ca^{2+} from the apical to the basolateral pole (see above). This restricts the degree to which Ca^{2+} mobilization at the apical pole can activate the basolateral K^+ channels. Might this restrict the efficacy of a therapy that relies upon apical purinergic activation? The answer, fortunately, is that this is probably not a serious issue. Ion fluxes across the apical membrane of airway epithelial cells are additionally subject to localized control processes. A key player is the apical Na^+ channel (ENaC).

The electrogenic uptake of Na^+ into the cell through ENaC is electrically coupled to Cl⁻ exit across the apical membrane through CFTR and CaCC.[20] Indeed, the Cl- efflux through CFTR normally down-regulates Na+ accumulation.[21-23] Thus, the CF defect is not only a reflection of a loss of Cl⁻ secretion, but in addition, the accompanying enhanced Na^+ absorption contributes to the pathophysiology of the CF lung disease.[23] However, inhibitors of ENaC, such as amiloride, have not yet been proven to be therapeutically useful in the treatment of CF.[2] On the other hand, activation of apical purinergic receptors in polarized CF cells not only enhances CaCC, but also inhibits EnaC.[22,24] In fact, this inhibition of ENaC by purinergic agonists is sufficiently striking that it might not be explained purely by electrical coupling between Na^+ uptake by ENaC and Cl⁻ efflux through CaCC.[22] Other molecular processes may be involved that merit further exploration.[22]

Several studies have indicated that chloride secretion triggered by apical $P2Y_2$ receptor activation is up-regulated in CF airway epithelia, compared to normal cells. For example, a report utilizing double-barreled chloride selective microelectrodes in normal and CF nasal epithelia revealed that luminal ATP promoted a greater increase in chloride secretion and in an apical chloride conductance in CF compared to normal epithelia.[19] Consistent with the microelectrode data, *in vivo* measurements of ATP or UTP-dependent nasal electrical potential difference (PD) showed a two-fold greater response in CF patients than that observed in normal subjects.[25,26] A similar phenomenon was also observed in primary cultures of CF human nasal epithelia compared to cultures from normal individuals.[26] In part, the up-regulated CaCC activity in human CF airway epithelia is facilitated by an elevated Ca^{2+} signal compared to normal airway cells.[17] The same mechanism also appears to operate in murine airway epithelia.[27]

However, there are other differences between wild-type and CF cells that cannot be attributed to differences in cellular $[Ca^{2+}]$ levels. This conclusion arose from experiments with normal and CF mouse tracheal epithelial (MTE) cell lines. These models confirmed that there is a reciprocal relationship between CFTR and CaCC conductances.[28,27] However, it was found that the upregulation of CaCC in CF cells was absolutely dependent on cell polarity and that when cells were rapidly dissociated, this phenomenon was not observed. Thus, as in many secretion studies, the relevance of *in vitro* results to the situation *in vivo* depends upon the model cell system employed, and definitive characterization of epithelial cell channels requires the channels to be expressed in the most physiologically relevant system, i.e., a polarized confluent epithelial monolayer. In further experiments with the MTEs, the basolateral membrane was selectively permeabilized so as to prevent it from electrochemically influencing chloride conductance at the apical membran.[27] This model also facilitated experimental control over intracellular $[Ca^{2+}]$. It was concluded that there was an increase in inherent CaCC activity in the CF cells.[27] This could be explained by the CF cells either having more Ca^{2+}-activated Cl^- channels, or their open probability might increase. Single channel analyses may resolve this issue.

4. PERSISTENT ACTIVATION OF PLC AS A CF THERAPY: THE PROBLEM OF INS(3,4,5,6)P$_4$

Control over a physiological process can be tuned to an especially fine extent by its regulation through a balance between signals with opposing influences. Control over CaCC by inositol phosphates provides an example of a regulatory process that operates through a dynamic balance between stimulatory and inhibitory signals. Receptor-activated, PLC-mediated increases in cellular Ins(1,4,5)P$_3$ levels are inevitably coupled to increases in Ins(3,4,5,6)P$_4$ levels.[29,30] The significance of this lies in the fact that Ins(3,4,5,6)P$_4$ is an inhibitor of CaCC.[5,6,31-33] This phenomenon has been demonstrated using three different model systems: Cl^- secretion from polarized epithelial monolayers was inhibited by cell-permeant analogues of Ins(3,4,5,6)P$_4$;[4,34] CaCC was inhibited in whole-cell patch-clamp experiments when Ins(3,4,5,6)P$_4$ was introduced into the cell interior;[5,6,31] recombinant CaCC incorporated into lipid bilayers was blocked by Ins(3,4,5,6)P$_4$.[33] Thus, the efficacy of persistent or repetitive activation of PLC as a therapy for CF is constrained by the fact that the accompanying elevated levels of Ins(3,4,5,6)P$_4$ have the capacity to inhibit the very channels that the therapy is designed to activate. This effect of Ins(3,4,5,6)P$_4$ is highly-specific, and is not imitated by any other inositol phosphates normally found inside cells, such as Ins(1,3,4,5,6)P$_5$, Ins(1,4,5,6)P$_4$, Ins(1,3,4,5)P$_4$, Ins(1,3,4,6)P$_4$, Ins(1,4,5)P$_3$ or Ins(1,3,4)P$_3$.[5,31,6]

How are PLC-mediated increases in Ins(1,4,5)P$_3$ levels coupled to elevations in Ins(3,4,5,6)P$_4$ concentrations? Ins(1,4,5)P$_3$ metabolism, through mass action effects, leads to accompanying increases in many downstream metabolites. In some cells, this "metabolic domino" effect may stretch as far as Ins(3,4,5,6)P$_4$ (i.e. Ins(1,4,5)P$_3$ -> Ins(1,3,4,5)P$_4$ -> Ins(1,3,4)P$_3$ -> Ins(1,3,4,6)P$_4$ -> Ins(1,3,4,5,6)P$_5$ -> Ins(3,4,5,6)P$_4$). However, in most cases it appears this is not the major mechanism by which Ins(3,4,5,6)P$_4$ levels are regulated. This conclusion arose after it was demonstrated that Ins(3,4,5,6)P$_4$ [and Ins(1,3,4,5,6)P$_5$] belong to a metabolic pool that is separate from that of Ins(1,4,5)P$_3$ and its more closely-related metabolites.[35,36] In other words, in the short-term, the metabolic pool of

$Ins(3,4,5,6)P_4$ is somewhat insulated from changes in $Ins(1,4,5)P_3$ concentrations. This phenomenon is clearly seen during short-term radiolabelling of cells with [^3H]inositol; $Ins(1,4,5)P_3$ equilibrates with radiolabel much faster than does $Ins(3,4,5,6)P_4$.[35] It is also relevant to this hypothesis that there are circumstances where a receptor-dependent *increase* in $Ins(3,4,5,6)P_4$ levels is associated with a *decrease* in $Ins(1,3,4,5,6)P_5$ levels.[35] The latter phenomenon clearly cannot result from a mass-action relationship between $Ins(1,3,4,5,6)P_5$ and $Ins(3,4,5,6)P_4$. Instead, there are other receptor-dependent mechanisms that can directly regulate $Ins(3,4,5,6)P_4$ metabolism. A central feature of this process is the closed metabolic cycle that interconverts $Ins(3,4,5,6)P_4$ and $Ins(1,3,4,5,6)P_5$ through the actions of an $Ins(3,4,5,6)P_4$ 1-kinase and an $Ins(1,3,4,5,6)P_5$ 1-phosphatase activities. In a series of studies [30,37,38] it has been demonstrated that $Ins(1,3,4)P_3$ competitively inhibits the activity of the $Ins(3,4,5,6)P_4$ 1-kinase. This changes the poise of the closed $Ins(3,4,5,6)P_4$ 1-kinase / $Ins(1,3,4,5,6)P_5$ 1-phosphatase substrate cycle. Thus, $Ins(3,4,5,6)P_4$ levels inevitably become elevated in response to an accumulation of $Ins(1,3,4)P_3$. Since elevations in $Ins(1,3,4)P_3$ levels accompany PLC activation, this sequence of events explains the link between receptor-mediated PLC activation, and increases in $Ins(3,4,5,6)P_4$ levels.

Experiments with recombinant human $Ins(3,4,5,6)P_4$ 1-kinase revealed that $Ins(1,3,4)P_3$ inhibits the enzyme because $Ins(1,3,4)P_3$ is a competing substrate.[39] This observation may initially seem puzzling, because, unlike $Ins(3,4,5,6)P_4$, the $Ins(1,3,4)P_3$ does not have a free 1-hydroxyl to be phosphorylated. However, we should not always compare the structures of two inositol phosphates in the same orientation. If instead $Ins(1,3,4)P_3$ is flipped upside down and rotated, some structural resemblance to $Ins(3,4,5,6)P_4$ becomes evident (see ref40 for a detailed description). In this comparison, four groups attached to the inositol ring of $Ins(3,4,5,6)P_4$, namely, the 1-OH, 3-phosphate, 4-phosphate and 6-phosphate, all have surrogates in $Ins(1,3,4)P_3$: respectively, the 6-OH, 4-phosphate, 3-phosphate and 1-phosphate. In particular, the 1-OH in $Ins(3,4,5,6)P_4$ that is phosphorylated is equivalent to the 6-OH in $Ins(1,3,4)P_3$.

Both $Ins(1,3,4)P_3$ and $Ins(3,4,5,6)P_4$ are phosphorylated by this kinase with similar K_m and V_{max} values.[39] It follows that the metabolic rivalry between $Ins(3,4,5,6)P_4$ and $Ins(1,3,4)P_3$ for phosphorylation by the 1-/6-kinase is most intense, and therefore of significance to the regulation of $Ins(3,4,5,6)P_4$ levels, if the concentrations of both substrates are also similar *in vivo*.[30,39] This appears to be the case: $Ins(3,4,5,6)P_4$ levels fluctuate between 1 and 10 μM.[34,41] $Ins(1,3,4)P_3$ levels have also been placed in this low micromolar range.[42-44] PLC-dependent increases in $Ins(1,3,4)P_3$ therefore inhibit Ins(3,4,5,6)P$_4$ phosphorylation, which then increases in concentration.

It was recently noted that there is something rather more complex about the mechanism of Ins(1,3,4)P$_3$ action that goes beyond mere competitive inhibition of Ins(3,4,5,6)P$_4$ 1-kinase activity. It has been recently discovered that the Ins(3,4,5,6)P$_4$ 1-kinase is physiologically reversible.[45] That is, the enzyme also acts as an Ins(1,3,4,5,6)P$_5$ 1-phosphatase.[45] This property initially emerged after recombinant human enzyme was incubated with ADP and Ins(1,3,4,5,6)P$_5$.[45] Of course, in principle, any phosphokinase is reversible if the ADP/ATP ratio is sufficiently high. However, it has been demonstrated that the enzyme does operate as an Ins(1,3,4,5,6)P$_5$ 1-phosphatase *in vivo*: T$_{84}$ cells were stably transfected with the enzyme, which prompted an amplification of receptor-dependent increases in Ins(3,4,5,6)P$_4$ levels.[45] It further appeared from *in vitro* studies that Ins(1,3,4)P$_3$ accelerates the rate of Ins(1,3,4,5,6)P$_5$ dephosphorylation.[45] The underlying mechanism is still unclear, but one possibility is that the 1-phosphate that is cleaved from Ins(1,3,4,5,6)P$_5$ can be transferred to Ins(3,4,5,6)P$_4$.[45] The multifunctional nature of the reversible kinase/phosphatase would seem likely to require the operation of more than one ligand-binding domain. The structure of the enzyme has not yet been solved, but the available evidence points to there only being a single catalytic site within this 46 kDa protein.[40] It is possible that, *in vivo*, the protein acquires more than one catalytic domain by oligomerization, perhaps driven by domain swapping.[46] Further experiments are required in order to examine these ideas.

These data described above have raised the possibility that if it were possible to pharmacologically or genetically manipulate CaCC regulation by the Ins(3,4,5,6)P$_4$-signaling pathway, this might provide a novel therapeutic approach to CF. For example, it may be possible to decrease the expression of the Ins(1,3,4,5,6)P$_5$ phosphatase activity that generates Ins(3,4,5,6)P$_4$. Such an experimental approach has yet to be attempted, although the converse experiment confirms a genetic approach to the manipulation of Ins(3,4,5,6)P$_4$ levels is feasible. That is, over-expression of Ins(1,3,4,5,6)P$_5$ phosphatase activity increased Ins(3,4,5,6)P$_4$ levels and reduced Cl$^-$ secretion across epithelial monolayers.[45] Unfortunately, we have to bear in mind that the Ins(1,3,4,5,6)P$_5$ 1-phosphatase is also the Ins(1,3,4)P$_3$ 6-kinase;[45] the latter activity is required for adequate synthesis of InsP$_6$ and the functionally-important diphosphorylated inositolphosphates.[40] Thus, non-specific cellular effects can arise from efforts to manipulate the expression of Ins(3,4,5,6)P$_4$ kinase / Ins(1,3,4,5,6)P$_5$ 1-phosphatase activity. In a different approach, other investigators have developed cell-permeant analogues of Ins(3,4,5,6)P$_4$ that can antagonize Ins(3,4,5,6)P$_4$-mediated inhibition of Cl⁻ secretion from epithelial monolayers.[7] It has also been shown that inhibition of Ser/Thr protein phosphatase activity is extremely effective at preventing $Ins(3,4,5,6)P_4$ from inhibiting CaCC.[5,32] In theory at least, this presents an alternate strategy to antagonize $Ins(3,4,5,6)P_4$, although it will be a challenge to develop a protein phosphatase inhibitor that specifically targets the $Ins(3,4,5,6)P_4$ signaling system and not the huge range of other actions of Ser/Thr phosphatases.

It must also be taken into account that the airways of CF null transgenic mice exhibit a much less severe pathology than that seen in humans.[47,48] One possible explanation for this lack of pathology is that CaCC is a much less active pathway for apical Cl⁻ exit in the human airway, compared to the mouse model. If the explanation is that relatively few ion channels that mediate CaCC are present in the human airway cells, this would present a particularly difficult challenge to PLC activation as a therapeutic approach.

However, an alternate possibility is that a therapeutically-useful number of CaCC proteins do exist in human airway cells, but their activity could be constitutively constrained. There is actually evidence in the literature which lends support to this idea. Data on the efficacy of $Ins(3,4,5,6)P_4$ as a CaCC inhibitor can be used to divide these channels into two distinct categories. One group are unaffected by 1 μM $Ins(3,4,5,6)P_4$, which is approximately the level of this cellular signal observed in unstimulated cells.[30] These channels only become inhibited by $Ins(3,4,5,6)P_4$ after PLC activation, whereupon levels of this inositol phosphate are elevated 4-10 fold.[5,31,6] The molecular identity of these particular channels is uncertain. However, a different group of CaCC, which have been cloned,[49] are blocked by as little as 20-200 nM $Ins(3,4,5,6)P_4$.[50,33] If these data are physiologically relevant, it must be concluded that these channels are constitutively inhibited even by the levels of $Ins(3,4,5,6)P_4$ prevailing in unstimulated cells. These particular channels are more widely known by their CLCA acronym. The human type 2 and type 3 species of CLCA are reportedly expressed in airway epithelia.[12,51,52] The possibility that these particular channels might be especially amenable to de-inhibition by $Ins(3,4,5,6)P_4$ antagonists merits further exploration.

5.   CONCLUSIONS

In this review, we have presented the mechanisms by which purinergic agonists activate CaCC. We have also paid particular attention to the polarization of the signaling processes that regulate CaCC. Current studies in our laboratories are under way to address whether additional components of the PLC-dependent apical membrane restricted regulation of CaCC are also confined to the apical pole of airway epithelia, e.g., Ins(1,4,5)P$_3$-sensitive ER Ca^{2+} stores and key enzymes involved in the metabolism of Ins(3,4,5,6)P$_4$. These studies should advance our understanding of the regulation of CaCC and may provide new clues to therapeutic procedures that might improve CaCC-dependent Cl$^-$ secretion into the airways of CF patients. We have described a new strategy for activating CaCC, based on the idea that drugs could be developed to antagonize Ins(3,4,5,6)P$_4$-mediated inhibition of CaCC.

There is as yet, little optimism that a single "wonder drug" could be developed that will restore lung function to CF individuals.[2] However, it does now seem realistic to hope that we might at least decrease the rate of lung deterioration with a combinatorial approach that utilizes several drugs that work in a co-operative manner.[2] For example, a PLC activator could be combined with an Ins(3,4,5,6)P$_4$ antagonist and an ENaC inhibitor. It is this approach to CF therapy that we propose can be served by intervention in the inositol phosphate signaling pathway.

REFERENCES

1. D. Kellerman, R. Evans, D. Mathews, and C. Shaffer, Inhaled P2Y2 receptor agonists as a treatment for patients with Cystic Fibrosis lung disease, *Adv. Drug Deliv. Rev.* **54**, 1463-1474 (2002).
2. G. M. Roomans Pharmacological approaches to correcting the ion transport defect in cystic fibrosis, *Am. J. Respir. Med.* **2**, 413-431 (2003).
3. B. R. Yerxa, J. R. Sabater, C. W. Davis, M. J. Stutts, M. Lang-Furr, M. Picher, A. C. Jones, M. Cowlen, R. Dougherty, J. Boyer, W. M. Abraham, and R. C. Boucher, Pharmacology of INS37217 [P(1)-(uridine 5')-P(4)- (2'-deoxycytidine 5')tetraphosphate, tetrasodium salt], a next-generation P2Y(2) receptor agonist for the treatment of cystic fibrosis, *J. Pharmacol. Exp. Ther.* **302**, 871-880 (2002).
4. M. A. Carew, X. Yang, C. Schultz, and S. B. Shears, Ins(3,4,5,6)P4 inhibits an apical calcium-activated chloride conductance in polarized monolayers of a cystic fibrosis cell-line, *J. Biol. Chem.* **275**, 26906-26913 (2000).
5. M. W. Y. Ho, M. A. Kaetzel, D. L. Armstrong, and S. B. Shears, Regulation of a Human Chloride Channel: A Paradigm for Integrating Input from Calcium, CaMKII and Ins(3,4,5,6)P4., *J. Biol. Chem.* **276**, 18673-18680 (2001).
6. W. Xie, M. A. Kaetzel, K. S. Bruzik, J. R. Dedman, S. B. Shears, and D. J. Nelson, Inositol 3,4,5,6-tetrakisphosphate inhibits the calmodulin-dependent protein kinase II-activated chloride conductance inT84 colonic epithelial cells, *J. Biol. Chem.* **271**, 14092-14097 (1996).
7. M. T. Rudolf, C. Dinkel, A. E. Traynor-Kaplan, and C. Schultz, Antagonists of myo-inositol 3,4,5,6-tetrakisphosphate allow repeated epithelial chloride secretion, *Bioorgan. Med. Chem.* **11**, 3315-3329 (2003).
8. H. A. Brown, E. R. Lazarowski, R. C. Boucher, and T. K. Harden, Evidence that UTP and ATP regulate phospholipase C through a common extracellular 5'-nucleotide receptor in human airway epithelial cells, *Mol. Pharmacol.* **40**, 648-655 (1991).

9. J. W. Putney, Jr., A model for receptor-regulated calcium entry, *Cell Calcium* **7**, 1-12 (1986).
10. J. W. Putney, Jr., Capacitative calcium entry revisited, *Cell Calcium* **11**, 611-624 (1991).
11. D. E. Clapham, Intracellular calcium. Replenishing the stores, *Nature* **375**, 634-635 (1995).
12. M. Mall, T. Gonska, J. Thomas, R. Schreiber, H. H. Seydewitz, J. Kuehr, M. Brandis, and K. Kunzelmann, Modulation of Ca2+-activated Cl- secretion by basolateral K+ channels in human normal and cystic fibrosis airway epithelia, *Pediatr. Res.* **53**, 608-618 (2003).
13. O. H. Petersen Stimulus-secretion coupling: cytoplasmic calcium signals and the control of ion channels in exocrine acinar cells, *J. Physiol.* (Lond.) **448**, 1-51 (1992).
14. T. Begenisich and J. E. Melvin, Regulation of chloride channels in secretory epithelia, *J. Membr. Biol.* **163**, 77-85 (1998).
15. V. L. Cressman, E. Lazarowski, L. Homolya, R. C. Boucher, B. H. Koller, and B. R. Grubb, Effect of loss of P2Y(2) receptor gene expression on nucleotide regulation of murine epithelial Cl(-) transport, *J. Biol. Chem.* **274**, 26461-26468 (1999).
16. A. M. Paradiso, S. J. Mason, E. R. Lazarowski, and R. C. Boucher, Membrane-restricted regulation of Ca2+ release and influx in polarized epithelia, *Nature* **377**, 643-646 (1995).
17. A. M. Paradiso, C. M. P. Ribeiro, and R. C. Boucher, Polarized signaling via purinoceptors in normal and cystic fibrosis airway epithelia, *J. Gen. Physiol.* **117**, 53-67 (2001).
18. C. M. Ribeiro, A. M. Paradiso, A. Livraghi, and R. C. Boucher, The Mitochondrial Barriers Segregate Agonist-induced Calcium-dependent Functions in Human Airway Epithelia, *J. Gen. Physiol.* **122**, 377-387 (2003).
19. L. L. Clarke and R. C. Boucher, Chloride secretory response to extracellular ATP in human normal and cystic fibrosis nasal epithelia, *Am. J. Physiol.* **263**, C348-C356 (1992).
20. J. D. Horisberger, ENaC-CFTR interactions: the role of electrical coupling of ion fluxes explored in an epithelial cell model, *Pflugers Arch.* **445**, 522-528 (2003).
21. R. C. Boucher, C. U. Cotton, J. T. Gatzy, M. R. Knowles, and J. R. Yankaskas, Evidence for reduced Cl- and increased Na+ permeability in cystic fibrosis human primary cell cultures, *J. Physiol.* **405**, 77-103 (1988).
22. D. C. Devor and J. M. Pilewski, UTP inhibits Na+ absorption in wild-type and ☐F508 CFTR-expressing human bronchial epithelia, *Am. J. Physiol.* **276**, C827-C837 (1999).
23. K. Kunzelmann ENaC is inhibited by an increase in the intracellular Cl(-) concentration mediated through activation of Cl(-) channels, *Pflugers Arch.* **445**, 504-512 (2003).
24. M. Mall, A. Wissner, T. Gonska, D. Calenborn, J. Kuehr, M. Brandis, and K. Kunzelmann, Inhibition of amiloride-sensitive epithelial Na(+) absorption by extracellular nucleotides in human normal and cystic fibrosis airways, *Am. J. Respir. Cell Mol. Biol.* **23** 755-761 (2000).
25. M. R. Knowles, L. L. Clarke, and R. C. Boucher, Extracellular ATP and UTP induce chloride secretion in nasal epithelia of Cystic Fibrosis patients and normal subjects in vivo, *Chest* **101**, 60S-63S (1992).
26. M. R. Knowles, L. L. Clarke, and R. C. Boucher, Activation by extracellular nucleotides of chloride secretion in the airway epithelial cells of patients with cystic fibrosis, *N. Engl. J. Med.* **325**, 533-538 (1991).
27. R. Tarran, M. E. Loewen, A. M. Paradiso, J. C. Olsen, M. A. Gray, B. E. Argent, R. C. Boucher, and S. E. Gabriel, Regulation of murine airway surface liquid volume by CFTR and Ca2+-activated Cl- conductances, *J. Gen. Physiol.* **120**, 407-418 (2002).
28. S. E. Gabriel, M. Makhlina, E. Martsen, E. J. Thomas, M. I. Lethem, and R. C. Boucher, Permeabilization via the P2X7 purinoreceptor reveals the presence of a Ca2+-activated Cl-

conductance in the apical membrane of murine tracheal epithelial cells, *J. Biol. Chem.* **275**, 35028-35033 (2000).

29. M. W. Y. Ho and S. B. Shears, Regulation of calcium-activated chloride channels by inositol 3,4,5,6-tetrakisphosphate, *Curr. Top. Membr.* **53**, 345-363 (2002)

30. Z. Tan, K. S. Bruzik, and S. B. Shears, Properties of the inositol 3,4,5,6-tetrakisphosphate 1-kinase purified from rat liver. Regulation of enzyme activity by inositol 1,3,4-trisphosphate, *J. Biol. Chem.* **272**, 2285-2290 (1997).

31. M. W. Y. Ho, S. B. Shears, K. S. Bruzik, M. Duszyk, and A. S. French, Inositol 3,4,5,6-tetrakisphosphate specifically inhibits a receptor-mediated Ca2+-dependent Cl- current in CFPAC-1 cells, *Am. J. Physiol.* **272**, C1160-C1168 (1997).

32. W. Xie, K. R. H. Solomons, S. Freeman, M. A. Kaetzel, K. S. Bruzik, D. J. Nelson, and S. B. Shears, Regulation of Ca^{2+}-dependent Cl^- conductance in T84 cells: cross-talk between Ins(3,4,5,6)P$_4$ and protein phosphatases, *J. Physiol.*(Lond.) **510**, 661-673 (1998).

33. I. I. Ismailov, C. M. Fuller, B. K. Berdiev, V. G. Shlyonsky, D. J. Benos, and K. E. Barrett, A biologic function for an "orphan" messenger: D-myo-Inositol 3,4,5,6-tetrakisphosphate selectively blocks epithelial calcium-activated chloride current, *Proc. Natl. Acad. Sci. U.S.A.* **93**, 10505-10509 (1996).

34. M. Vajanaphanich, C. Schultz, M. T. Rudolf, M. Wasserman, P. Enyedi, A. Craxton, S. B. Shears, R. Y. Tsien, K. E. Barrett, and A. E. Traynor-Kaplan, Long-term uncoupling of chloride secretion from intracellular calcium levels by Ins(3,4,5,6)P$_4$, *Nature* **371**, 711-714 (1994).

35. F. S. Menniti, K. G. Oliver, K. Nogimori, J. F. Obie, S. B. Shears, and J. W. Putney, Jr., Origins of myo-inositol tetrakisphosphates in agonist-stimulated rat pancreatoma cells. Stimulation by bombesin of myo-inositol 1,3,4,5,6-pentakisphosphate breakdown to myo-inositol 3,4,5,6-tetrakisphosphate, *J. Biol. Chem.* **265**, 11167-11176 (1990).

36. N. S. Wong, C. J. Barker, A. J. Morris, A. Craxton, C. J. Kirk, and R. H. Michell, The inositol phosphates of WRK1 rat mammary tumour cells, *Biochem. J.* **286**, 459-468 (1992).

37. X. Yang, M. Rudolf, M. Yoshida, M. A. Carew, A. M. Riley, S.-K. Chung, K. S. Bruzik, B. V. L. Potter, C. Schultz, and S. B. Shears, Ins(1,3,4)P$_3$ acts in vivo as a specific regulator of cellular signaling by Ins(3,4,5,6)P$_4$, *J. Biol. Chem.* **274**, 18973-18980 (1999).

38. A. Craxton, C. Erneux, and S. B. Shears, Inositol 1,4,5,6-tetrakisphosphate is phosphorylated in rat liver by a 3-kinase that is distinct from inositol 1,4,5-trisphosphate 3-kinase, *J. Biol. Chem.* **269**, 4337-4342 (1994).

39. X. Yang and S. B. Shears, Multitasking in Signal Transduction by a Promiscuous Human Ins(3,4,5,6)P$_4$ 1-Kinase/Ins(1,3,4)P3 5/6-Kinase, *Biochem. J.* **351**, 551-555 (2000).

40. S. B. Shears, How versatile are inositol phosphate kinases? *Biochem. J.* **377**, 265-280 (2004).

41. D. Pittet, W. Schlegel, D. P. Lew, A. Monod, and G. W. Mayr, Mass changes in inositol tetrakis- and pentakisphosphate isomers induced by chemotactic peptide stimulation in HL-60 cells, *J. Biol. Chem.* **264**, 18489-18493 (1989).

42. P. J. Hughes, A. R. Hughes, J. W. Putney, Jr., and S. B. Shears, The regulation of the phosphorylation of inositol (1,3,4)-trisphosphate in cell free preparations and its relevance to the formation of inositol (1,3,4,6)-tetrakisphosphate in agonist-stimulated rat parotid acinar cells, *J. Biol. Chem.* **264**, 19871-19878 (1989).

43. A. P. Tarver, W. G. King, and S. E. Rittenhouse, Inositol 1,4,5-trisphosphate and inositol 1,2-cyclic 4,5-trisphosphate are minor components of total mass of inositol trisphosphate in thrombin-stimulated platelets, *J. Biol. Chem.* **262**, 17268-17271 (1987).

44. G. Li, W.-F. Pralong, D. Pittet, G. W. Mayr, W. Schlegel, and C. B. Woolheim, Inositol tetrakisphosphate isomers and elevation of cytosolic calcium in vasopressin-stimulated insulin-secreting RINm5F cells, *J. Biol. Chem.* **267**, 4349-4356 (1992).
45. M. Y. H. Ho, X. Yang, M. A. Carew, T. Zhang, L. Hua, Y.-U. Kwon, S.-K. Chung, S. Adelt, G. Vogel, A. M. Riley, B. V. L. Potter, and S. B. Shears, Regulation of Ins(3456)P$_4$ signaling by a reversible kinase/phosphatase, *Current Biology* **12**, 477-482 (2002).
46. Y. Liu and D. Eisenberg, 3D domain swapping: As domains continue to swap, *Protein science* **11**, 1285-1299 (2002).
47. B. R. Grubb and R. C. Boucher, Pathophysiology of gene-targeted mouse models for cystic fibrosis, *Physiol. Rev.* **79**, S193-S214 (1999).
48. J. N. Snouwaert, K. K. Brigman, A. M. Latour, R. C. Boucher, O. Smithies, and B. H. Koller, An animal model for cystic fibrosis made by gene targeting., *Science* **257**, 1083-1088 (1992).
49. A. D. Gruber, R. C. Elbe, and B. U. Pauli, Cloning of the CLCA gene family, *Curr. Top. Membr.* **53**, 368-387 (2002).
50. H. Zhang, M. McCarthy, K. E. Barrett, J. R. Yankaskas, D. J. Benos, and C. M. Fuller, Ca^{2+}-activated Cl$^-$ conductances in normal and CF airway epithelia, *Ped. Pulm. Suppl.* **21**, A88 (2001).
51. A. D. Gruber, K. D. Schreur, H.-L. Ji, C. M. Fuller, and B. U. Pauli, Molecular cloning and transmembrane structure of hCLCA2 from human lung, trachea and mammary gland, *Am. J. Physiol.* **276**, C1261-C1270 (1999).
52. B. U. Pauli, M. Abdel-Ghany, H.-C. Cheng, A. D. Gruber, H. A. Archibald, and R. C. Elble, Molecular characteristics and functional diversity of CLCA family members, *Clin. Exp. Pharmacol. Physiol.* **27** 901-905 (2000).

Chapter 9

AN INOSITOL PHOSPHATE ANALOG, INO-4995, NORMALIZES ELECTROPHYSIOLOGY IN CF AIRWAY EPITHELIA

Alexis Traynor-Kaplan,[1] Mark Moody,[1] and Carsten Schultz[2]

[1]*Inologic Inc., 101 Elliott Ave. W., Seattle, 98119 WA, USA;* [2]*European Molecular Biology Laboratory, Meyerhofstr. 1, 69117 Heidelberg, Germany, e-mail: alexis@inologic.com*

1.   INTRODUCTION

In cystic fibrosis (CF) a combination of ion transport abnormalities results in a reduced capacity to control airway surface liquid volume resulting in viscous mucus that fosters bacterial growth leading to repeated infections, lung damage and ultimately organ failure.[1,2] CF is caused by mutations in the gene coding for the cystic fibrosis transmembrane conductance regulator (CFTR) protein resulting in defective Cl⁻ transport and disregulation of a host of apical ion channels. For instance, this defect is also linked to hyperabsorption of Na^+ through the epithelial Na^+ channel $(ENaC)^{3-5}$ that underlies the abnormal physiology characterized by elevated basal short circuit current (I_{sc}) and large potential difference (PD) in CF mucosal airway epithelia.

Traditional treatments for CF have focused on managing symptoms. Physically assisted therapies such as chest percussion and postural drainage help clear mucus secretions, while three medications are now available to alleviate symptoms. Two antibiotics, Tobi® and the more recently tested for efficacy in CF, Azithromycin, helps control infections. The other treatment on the market, Pulmozyme®, cleaves DNA strands from ruptured neutrophils to reduce excess mucus viscosity. While these agents provide relief for some CF sufferers and have helped extend the average lifespan to 33, they do not remedy the underlying defect. Consequently, novel approaches are still sought to extend life expectancy in CF patients. Current exploratory therapies are in various stages of preclinical and early clinical development and fall into broad categories that includes antibiotics, nutritional support, human stem cell therapy, anti-inflammatories, mucus regulation, gene therapy, CFTR protein rescue and ion channel modulators to normalize ion transport. Here we describe a novel method to normalize ion transport.

Efforts to rectify dysfunctional ion transport associated with CF have focused on modulating ENaC, CFTR, and alternate Cl⁻ channel function. There are compelling arguments for pursuing artificial activation of alternate Cl⁻ channels and regulation of ENaC to counteract CF pathophysiology.[6] Mucosal epithelia express Cl⁻ channels other than the CFTR such as the outwardly rectifying chloride channel (ORCC), calcium activated Cl⁻ channels (CLCA) and volume regulated Cl⁻ channels (ClCx) that are all potential targets for CF treatment. While the ORCC appears to be controlled by the CFTR and is thereby compromised in CF,[7-10] active CLCA channel activity is more abundant in CF tissue.[11] In fact phenotypes with increased CLCA activity correlate with milder clinical manifestations.[7,12-15] Stimulation of apical Cl⁻ secretion through the CFTR and CLCA channels is closely associated with ENaC function and Na⁺ absorption in mucosal epithelia.[5,16-19] Thus, alternate Cl⁻ channels such as the CLCA channel and the ClC-x family may compensate for defects in CFTR function and could be utilized in a therapeutic strategy. This idea has spawned a number of clinical trials. Recently, Sucampo pharmaceuticals began testing a prostaglandin analog, SPI-8811, which targets ClC-x channels for efficacy in CF. Two other compounds in development target CLCA by elevating intracellular Ca^{2+}, INS365, a PY2Y receptor agonist (Inspire Pharmaceuticals) and duramycin (Moli 1901). However, some of these latter results have been disappointing, presumably because of the inherent transience of Ca^{2+} signaling.

Furthermore, an increase in intracellular Ca^{2+} does not always lead to Cl⁻ secretion. We have demonstrated that the intracellular signaling molecule, *myo*-inositol 3,4,5,6-tetrakisphosphate [Ins(3,4,5,6)P₄] "uncouples" Cl⁻ secretion from the rise in intracellular Ca^{2+} in mucosal epithelia.[20,21] This regulatory role for Ins(3,4,5,6)P₄ has been confirmed by several investigators in various tissues including a CF pancreatic epithelial cell line, CFPAC-1.[22-26] Therefore, we hypothesized that antagonistic analogs of Ins(3,4,5,6)P₄ may stimulate CLCA. Such molecules would be expected to act "downstream" of the rise in intracellular Ca^{2+}. To test this we constructed a series of Ins(3,4,5,6)P₄ analogs and studied their effects in monolayer cultures of primary CF human nasal epithelial cells that exhibit many *in vivo* characteristics of CF mucosal epithelia. Since Ins(3,4,5,6)P₄ and constructed analogs are not membrane-permeant we masked the charged groups of these compounds with bioactivatable, lipophilic groups, that enable cell entry.[21,27]

Once inside, the masking groups are removed and the resulting Ins(3,4,5,6)P_4 derivatives may compete for Ins(3,4,5,6)P_4 binding sites.

Elevated basal I_{sc} is a prominent characteristic of cultures of CF human nasal airway epithelia that distinguishes it from normal tissue and recent studies suggest that it is directly linked to pathophysiology of CF lung disease.[6] Although basal I_{sc} is largely driven by Na^+ channel activity (ENaC) it has been closely associated with both CFTR as well as flux through other Cl^- channels.[5,16-19] For example, CFTR inhibits sodium absorption through ENaC such that CF epithelia exhibit a 2-3 fold increase in sodium absorption relative to normal epithelia.[28] Moreover, CLC coexpression with ENaC in Xenopus oocytes inhibits ENaC activity[29] and lack of lung disease in CF mice has been attributed to enhanced CLCA activity relative to human lungs.[11] However, the mechanism for these effects of chloride channels on ENaC remains controversial. We chose to screen our compounds for efficacy in lowering basal I_{sc} because it is convenient to measure and is particularly relevant to CF pathophysiology.

2.   METHODS

2.1   Materials

Surgically excised nasal polyps were obtained from volunteers in collaboration with Dr. Bonnie Ramsey at Children's Hospital, Seattle. Informed consent was obtained prior to receiving tissue specimens. All protocols were in compliance with institutional guidelines and approved by the Institutional Review Board at Children's Hospital in Seattle. INO-4995, inositol polyphosphates, phosphate/PM and other membrane-permeant inositol polyphosphate analogs were obtained from SiChem GmbH, Germany. All other reagents were provided by Sigma-Aldrich unless otherwise indicated.

2.2   CF Human Nasal Epithelial (CFHNE) Cell Culture

Surgically obtained nasal polyps were transported on ice in a sterile container containing a 1:1 mixture of Dulbecco's modification of minimum essential medium Eagle and Ham's F-12 nutrient medium (DMEM/F-12) (Irvine Scientific, Santa Ana, CA) supplemented with 100 U/ml penicillin, 0.1 mg/ml streptomycin, 10 mM HEPES, and 2 mM L-glutamine. CF tissue was homozygous for the ΔF508 mutation. The tissue samples were washed (5X) by suspending in 40 ml of Joklik's modification of minimum essential medium eagle (JMEM) at 4°C, allowing the tissue to settle to the bottom of the tube, and aspirating the supernatant. The tissue was then transferred to JMEM containing 200 U/ml penicillin, 0.2 mg/ml streptomycin, 0.1 mg/ml gentamycin sulfate (Clonetics, San Diego, CA), and 0.1 μg/ml amphotericin-B (Clonetics), and 0.1% protease (Sigma), washed an additional 2X, suspended in 15 ml of JMEM in a 10 cm tissue culture dish, and incubated at 4°C for 24 hrs. The tissue samples were gently triturated, the connective tissue aseptically removed, and the remaining cell suspension centrifuged at 1000 rpm for 5 min. The supernatant was aspirated and pellet resuspended in 10ml JMEM with 0.025% trypsin-EDTA and allowed to incubate for 5 min. after which 10% fetal bovine serum (FBS) was added to deactivate the trypsin, and the cell suspension was centrifuged at 1000 rpm. The supernatant was aspirated and cell pellet resuspended in a proliferation media consisting of keratinocyte-serum free medium (KSFM)(Gibco-BRL, Grand Island, NY) containing 5 ng/ml EGF (Gibco), 50 μg/ml BPE (Gibco), 100 U/ml penicillin, 0.1 mg/ml streptomycin, and 2 mM L-glutamine. The cell suspension was transferred to two 10 cm tissue culture dishes coated with 1 μg/cm^2 Vitrogen (Becton-Dickinson, Bedford, MA), incubated at 37°C in an humidified atmosphere of 5% CO_2 and 95% air. The cells were 70-80% confluent after 6 days with the media being replaced with every other day. The cells were then trypsinized using 0.025% trypsin-EDTA for 5 min. The cell suspension was collected, the trypsin deactivated with 10% FBS, and centrifuged at 1000 rpm for 5min. Cell counts were determined by hemocytometer. There was a typical yield of 3-4 x 10^6 cells per dish. The cells (passage 1) were then cryopreserved for future experiments. Passage 1 cells thawed from cryovials were cultured until they reached 90% confluence when they were trypsinized and plated on permeable supports (passage 2) (snapwells).

2.3   Monolayer Preparation for Ussing studies

Epithelial cells (passages 2 or 3) were prepared for Ussing Chamber and fluid transport studies using *Snapwell* permeable supports (0.4 μm pore size) (Corning Costar, Cambridge, MA) coated with 1 μg/cm^2 Vitrogen. Cells were plated at 10^5 cells/cm^2 in KSFM. After 2 days, the media was changed to bronchial epithelial growth medium (BEGM)(a 1:1 mixture of DMEM (MediaTech/Cellgro, Herndon, VA) and bronchial epithelial basal media (BEBM) (Clonetics/Biowhittaker, Walkersville, MD), with the following supplements: hydrocortisone (0.5 μg/ml), insulin (5 μg/ml), transferrin (10 μg/ml), epinephrine (0.5 μg/ml), triiodothyronine (6.5 ng/ml), bovine pituitary extract (52 μg/ml), EGF (0.5 ng/ml), all-*trans* retinoic acid (50 nM, Sigma), penicillin (100 U/ml, Sigma), streptomycin (0.1 mg/ml, Sigma), non-essential amino acids (1X, Sigma), and bovine serum albumin (fatty acid-free, 3 μg/ml, Sigma). Cells were grown in the BEGM for 1 week, at which point an air-liquid interface (ALI) culture system was initiated.[30] The cells were grown for 2 weeks at ALI, fed every other day basolaterally until use in the Ussing chamber (usually 7-10 days).

2.4   Ussing Chamber Studies

Monolayers of CFHNE were mounted in modified Ussing chambers (Physiologic Instruments, San Diego, CA) using Ringers bicarbonate solution containing (in mM): 115 NaCl, 2.4 K_2HPO_4 0.4 KH_2PO_4, 1.2 $MgCl_2$, 1.2 $CaCl_2$, 25 $NaHCO_3$, 10 glucose; unless otherwise indicated. Experiments were carried out at 37°C and the pH adjusted to 7.4 by gassing with 95%O_2/5%CO_2. After an open-circuit equilibration period of 10 min, the transepithelial PD was recorded and the monolayers were voltage clamped at 0 mV and the resulting I_{sc} was continuously recorded. A periodic bipolar voltage pulse monitored resistance calculated using Ohm's Law. In acute experiments, drugs were added to the apical or basolateral compartment, as indicated, and the changes in response recorded.   In preincubation experiments, compound dissolved in 100 μl of Ringers was added to the apical surface of monolayers growing on snapwells. After a 2 hour incubation at 37°C in a CO_2 incubator, the apical media with compound was removed, monolayers were washed with BEGM and returned to ALI for indicated time prior to mounting in Ussing chambers.

3.   RESULTS

3.1   Acute effect of INO-4995 on amiloride-inhibitable I_{sc}

The effect of INO-4995 on the electrical properties of monolayers of human CF nasal epithelia was tested in Ussing chambers.   The results depicted in Figure 1-3 show that adding 5 μM INO-4995 to the apical compartment of Ussing chambers results in a decline of I_{sc} leading to baseline over 100 minutes. This effect is not observed in monolayers treated similarly with INO-4949, an unesterified analog of INO-4995 or with the enantiomer of INO-4995, INO-4987. There was also a more gradual decline in monolayers that were not treated with compound which was not noticeably different from that of monolayers treated similarly with INO-4949, an unesterified analog of INO-4995 or with the enantiomer of INO-4995, INO-4987. Consistent with results of other investigators stimulation of purinergic receptors with 100 ATP increased I_{sc} when added after amiloride (Figure 1). However, 100 µM ATP caused a drop in basal Isc comparable to that caused by preincubation with 5 µM INO-4995 (Figure 2 and 3). Similar results have been described by other investigators who attributed the purinergic induced drop in I_{sc} to inhibition of ENaC.[17,19] Since we suspected the gradual decline in the non-treated monolayers was due in part to the prolonged time course necessary to see a full effect, we sought alternative protocols to minimize this artifact.

3.1.1   Peak effect and reversibility

As it took 1-2 hours to obtain a maximal inhibition of basal I_{sc} following acute addition of INO-4995 in our early experiments (Figures 1-3), we incubated monolayers for 2 hours with compound and then returned the monolayers to air liquid interface and incubated them for 24 hours before measuring their I_{sc} in Ussing chambers. This resulted in a stable dose-dependent inhibition of basal amiloride-inhibitable I_{sc} (Figure 4). These results demonstrated that the inhibition of I_{sc} with INO-4995 is long lasting but raised the question of whether the inhibitory effect was reversible. Hence we probed the duration of basal I_{sc} inhibition by measuring electrical

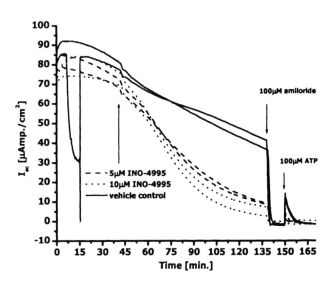

Figure 1. INO-4995 at the indicated doses and time was added to the apical compartment of Ussing chambers in which monolayers of primary CF human nasal epithelia (CFHNE) were mounted. Short circuit current (I_{sc}) was recorded. This experiment is representative of 5.

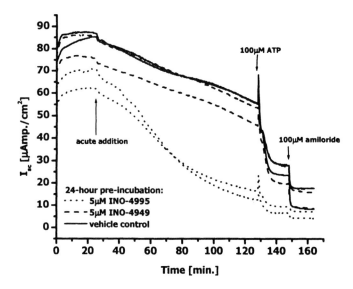

Figure 2. Comparison of the effect of INO-4995 and a de-esterified derivative, INO-4949 on basal I_{sc}.

properties including basal I_{sc} in Ussing chambers at 8, 24, 48, and 72 hours after a two hour incubation with INO-4995. The results showed that the effect of a 2 hour incubation with 5 μM INO-4995 was virtually unchanged between 8 hours and 24 hrs after incubation (Figure 5). At 24 hours post exposure INO-4995 still shows ~40% inhibition of basal I_{sc} relative to control values, comparable to inhibition observed at 8 hours. The effect was reversible, however, when treated monolayers were tested 48 and 72 hrs later (Figure 5). In fact by 48 hours the inhibitory effect of INO-4995 diminished to near control values. The data demonstrates that 5 μM INO-4995 reversibly inhibits I_{sc} for 22-48 hours (Figure 5).

In a separate experiment when monolayers were treated with 10 μM INO-4995 for 2 hours and I_{sc} tested 4 hours later, the degree of inhibition was comparable to the level of inhibition obtained with 10 μM INO-4995 at the 24 hour time point (data not shown) indicating that basal I_{sc} inhibition by INO-4995 remains near maximal levels for from 2 to at least 24 hours.

3.1.2   Optimizing incubation duration

In order to assess the rate of entry of compound into the cells, the duration of apical incubation with INO-4995 was varied from 30 min. to 4

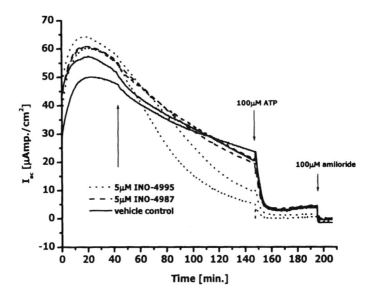

Figure 3. Comparison of the effect of INO-4995 with its enantiomer, INO-4987 on basal I_{sc} in CFHNE.

hrs. At respective times the buffer containing the compound or vehicle was removed and the monolayers returned to ALI culture. After 24 hrs from the time the compounds were first administered, the monolayers were mounted in Ussing chambers and the basal I_{sc} was measured.

While all incubations resulted in reduced I_{sc}, the major increase in potency occurred within the first 30-60 min, with no further change observed with longer incubations exceeding 60 min. (Figure 5).

4.   DISCUSSION

CF airway epithelia are characterized by accelerated sodium absorption and attenuated response to Cl⁻ secretagogues acting through cyclic AMP but not calcium pathways. Although Cl⁻ secretion in response to secretagogues is transient, the defect in sodium absorption is constant and detectable in cells that have not been exposed to triggering agents. In addition, while the impact of the Cl⁻ secretory defect may be more localized, the sodium absorption defect is observed consistently throughout the airway mucosal

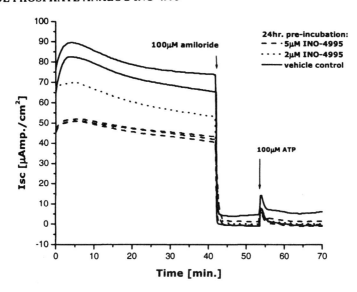

Figure 4. Comparison of the effect of 2 and 5 μM INO-4995 on amiloride-inhibitable I$_{sc}$ 24 h after a 2 h incubation with compound.

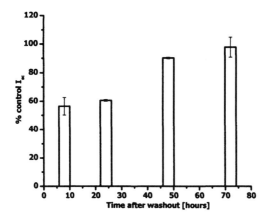

Figure 5. Time-dependent recovery of basal Isc inhibition following a single dose of 5mM INO-4995 (2 h exposure): Inhibition of basal Isc measured at 8, 24, 48, and 72 hours after exposure. Control=100%, n=11. Data calculated from the analysis of the Isc at 10min. Mean +/-SEM of the percent inhibition.

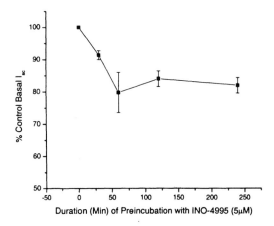

Figure 6. Effect of duration of preincubation with INO-4995 on its inhibition of basal I_{sc} in CF human nasal epithelia.

epithelia. Therefore, the defect in sodium absorption may be as relevant to CF pathophysiology as Cl^- secretion. For this reason, we focused our initial studies on the effect of INO-4995 on parameters directly linked to the sodium absorption defect, basal amiloride-inhibitable I_{sc} that was directly proportional to the initial potential difference (PD) across the monolayers.

Addition of INO-4995 directly to the apical compartment of Ussing chambers containing CF airway epithelia resulted in a slow decline of basal I_{sc} (Figures 1-3). This effect did not occur in monolayers exposed to a de-esterified form of the drug that would not be expected to cross the membrane and gain entry to the cell (Figure 2). In addition, an enantiomer of INO-4995 was without effect (Figure 3) demonstrating stereospecificity. The I_{sc} response to the drug is gradual, and complicated analysis of early studies. This lag time may reflect the kinetics of entry and de-esterification of the prodrug to the active drug inside the cell or it may reflect other processes set in motion following release of the de-esterified product inside the cell that are necessary for I_{sc} inhibition. Further complicating interpretation is the decline in I_{sc} in untreated monolayers possibly due to nutritional deficiencies in Ringers solution or to the periodic voltage pulses used to monitor resistance. Although these are potentially interesting questions to elucidate, we wanted to first characterize the physiological action of INO-4995 and identify a parameter that would be useful for dose/response analysis and comparison with other compounds. In order to circumvent some of the confounding variables, we exposed monolayers to compound for 2 hours in the incubator after which we returned the cells to air liquid interface culture and measured amiloride-inhibitable I_{sc} in Ussing chambers 22 hours later. This protocol resulted in a stable change in I_{sc} measurable at the 22-hour time point (Figure 4) that was more amenable to comparative analysis.

In addition, this demonstrated that INO-4995 could have a long lasting therapeutically relevant affect after a relatively brief exposure. We then sought to determine when the peak effect occurred and whether and over what time course the effect was reversible. The data depicted in Figure 5 indicate that a single 2 hour exposure to 5 µM INO-4995 reduces I_{sc} with little change for 8-22 hours after addition. Although some inhibition was still observable after 48 hours, basal I_{sc} completely returned to normal by 72 hours. In another experiment we saw no difference between a 4 and 24-hour incubation. Therefore, based on the kinetics of the effect shown in Figure 1 and the time course data, INO-4995 inhibition of basal I_{sc} reaches its peak within the first 2 hours of exposure and remains at this level for more than 22 hours.

We also questioned whether the duration of exposure might play a role in the magnitude of the inhibition. Longer exposures could result in diffusion of more prodrug into the cell and accumulation due to deesterification to the active drug. The data shown in Figure 6 demonstrate that the maximal effect is obtained with a one hour incubation when monolayers were incubated with 5 µM INO-4995 and that no further increase in efficacy was observed with longer incubations, presumably due to breakdown of compound in extracellular buffer after 1 hour incubation.

Based on these studies we can formulate an optimal experimental protocol for evaluating INO-4995 inhibition of basal I_{sc} and comparing its effects to other compounds.

5.   CONCLUSIONS

The effects of inositol polyphosphates on ion flux in CF mucosa described here suggest a novel therapeutic approach to the treatment of cystic fibrosis. These studies indicate that transient exposure to an inositol polyphosphate analog, INO-4995, causes long lasting but ultimately reversible changes in therapeutically relevant electrophysiological properties of CF human nasal epithelia. This avoids a major problem encountered with other ion channel regulators that have been advanced as potential CF treatments, limited duration of action.

REFERENCES

1. H. Matsui, B. R. Grubb, R. Tarran, S. H. Randell, J. T. Gatzy, C. W. Davis, and R. C. Boucher. Evidence for periciliary liquid layer depletion, not abnormal ion composition, in the pathogenesis of cystic fibrosis airways disease. *Cell* **95**, 1005-1015 (1998).
2. H. Matsui, C. W. Davis, R. Tarran, and R. C. Boucher. Osmotic water permeabilities of cultured, well-differentiated normal and cystic fibrosis airway epithelia, *J. Clin. Invest.* **105**, 1419-1427 (2000).
3. R. Greger. Role of CFTR in the colon, *Annu. Rev. Physiol.* **62**, 467-491 (2000).
4. R. C. Boucher, M. J. Stutts, M. R. Knowles, L. Cantley, and J. T. Gatzy. Na+ transport in cystic fibrosis respiratory epithelia. Abnormal basal rate and response to adenylate cyclase activation, *J. Clin. Invest.* **78**, 1245-1252 (1986).
5. M. Mall, M. Bleich, J. Kuehr, M. Brandis, R. Greger, and K. Kunzelmann. CFTR-mediated inhibition of epithelial Na+ conductance in human colon is defective in cystic fibrosis, *Am. J. Physiol.* **277**, G709-16 (1999).
6. M. R. Knowles and R. C. Boucher. Mucus clearance as a primary innate defense mechanism for mammalian airways, *J. Clin. Invest.* **109**, 571-577 (2002).
7. L. L. Clarke, B. R. Grubb, J. R. Yankaskas, C. U. Cotton, A. McKenzie, and R. C. Boucher. Relationship of a non-cystic fibrosis transmembrane conductance regulator-mediated chloride conductance to organ-level disease in Cftr(-/-) mice, *Proc. Natl. Acad. Sci. U.S.A.* **91**, 479-483 (1994).
8. S. E. Gabriel, L. L. Clarke, R. C. Boucher, and M. J. Stutts. CFTR and outward rectifying chloride channels are distinct proteins with a regulatory relationship, *Nature* **363**, 263-268 (1993).
9. M. Egan, T. Flotte, S. Afione, R. Solow, P. L. Zeitlin, B. J. Carter, and W. B. Guggino. Defective regulation of outwardly rectifying Cl- channels by protein kinase A corrected by insertion of CFTR. *Nature* **358**, 581-584 (1992).
10. E. M. Schwiebert, M. E. Egan, T. H. Hwang, S. B. Fulmer, S. S. Allen, G. R. Cutting, and W. B. Guggino. CFTR regulates outwardly rectifying chloride channels through an autocrine mechanism involving ATP. *Cell* **81**, 1063-1073 (1995).
11. B. R. Grubb, R. N. Vick, and R. C. Boucher. Hyperabsorption of Na+ and raised Ca(2+)-mediated Cl- secretion in nasal epithelia of CF mice, *Am. J. Physiol.* **266**, C1478-1483 (1994).
12. J. M. Pilewski and R. A. Frizzell. Role of CFTR in airway disease. *Physiol. Rev.* **79**, S215-255 (1999).
13. H. J. Veeze, D. J. Halley, J. Bijman, J. C. de Jongste, H. R. de Jonge, and M. Sinaasappel. Determinants of mild clinical symptoms in cystic fibrosis patients. Residual chloride secretion measured in rectal biopsies in relation to the genotype. *J. Clin. Invest.* **93**, 461-466 (1994).
14. A. Y. Leung, P. Y. Wong, S. E. Gabriel, J. R. Yankaskas, and R. C. Boucher. cAMP- but not Ca(2+)-regulated Cl⁻ conductance in the oviduct is defective in mouse model of cystic fibrosis. *Am. J. Physiol.* **268**, C708-712 (1995).
15. R. Rozmahel, M. Wilschanski, A. Matin, S. Plyte, M. Oliver, W. Auerbach, A. Moore, J. Forstner, P. Durie, J. Nadeau, C. Bear, and L. C. Tsui. Modulation of disease severity in cystic fibrosis transmembrane conductance regulator deficient mice by a secondary genetic factor. *Nat. Genet.* **12**, 280-287 (1996).
16. S. K. Inglis, A. Collett, H. L. McAlroy, S. M. Wilson, and R. E. Olver. Effect of luminal nucleotides on Cl- secretion and Na+ absorption in distal bronchi. *Pflugers Arch.* **438**, 621-627 (1999).

17. D. C. Devor and J. M. Pilewski. UTP inhibits Na+ absorption in wild-type and DeltaF508 CFTR-expressing human bronchial epithelia. *Am. J. Physiol.* **276**, C827-837 (1999).

18. S. J. Ramminger, D. L. Baines, R. E. Olver, and S. M. Wilson. The effects of PO2 upon transepithelial ion transport in fetal rat distal lung epithelial cells. *J. Physiol.* **524** Pt 2, 539-547 (2000).

19. X. F. Wang, and H. C. Chan. Adenosine triphosphate induces inhibition of Na(+) absorption in mouse endometrial epithelium: a Ca(2+)-dependent mechanism. *Biol. Reprod.* **63**, 1918-1924 (2000).

20. U. Kachintorn, M. Vajanaphanich, K. E. Barrett, and A. E. Traynor-Kaplan. Elevation of inositol tetrakisphosphate parallels inhibition of Ca(2+)-dependent Cl- secretion in T84 cells, *Am. J. Physiol.* **264**, C671-676 (1993).

21. M. Vajanaphanich, C. Schultz, M. T. Rudolf, M. Wasserman, P. Enyedi, A. Craxton, S. B. Shears, R. Y. Tsien, K. E. Barrett, and A. E. Traynor-Kaplan. Long-term uncoupling of chloride secretion from intracellular calcium levels by Ins(3,4,5,6)P$_4$. *Nature* **371**, 711-714 (1994).

22. M. W. Ho, S. B. Shears, K. S. Bruzik, M. Duszyk, and A. S. French. Ins(3,4,5,6)P$_4$ specifically inhibits a receptor-mediated Ca2+-dependent Cl- current in CFPAC-1 cells. *Am. J. Physiol.* **272**, C1160-1168 (1997).

23. W. Xie, K. R. Solomons, S. Freeman, M. A. Kaetzel, K. S. Bruzik, D. J. Nelson, and S. B. Shears. Regulation of Ca^{2+}-dependent Cl$^-$ conductance in a human colonic epithelial cell line (T84): cross-talk between Ins(3,4,5,6)P$_4$ and protein phosphatases. *J. Physiol.* **510**, 661-673 (1998).

24. I. I. Ismailov, C. M. Fuller, B. K. Berdiev, V. G. Shlyonsky, D. J. Benos, and K. E. Barrett. A biologic function for an "orphan" messenger: D-myo-inositol 3,4,5,6-tetrakisphosphate selectively blocks epithelial calcium-activated chloride channels. *Proc. Natl. Acad. Sci. U.S.A..* **93**, 10505-10509 (1996).

25. M. A. Carew and P. Thorn. Carbachol-stimulated chloride secretion in mouse colon: evidence of a role for autocrine prostaglandin E2 release. *Exp. Physiol.* **85**, 67-72 (2000).

26. M. A. Carew, X. Yang, C. Schultz, and S. B. Shears. myo-Inositol 3,4,5,6-tetrakisphosphate inhibits an apical calcium- activated chloride conductance in polarized monolayers of a cystic fibrosis cell line. *J. Biol. Chem.* **275**, 26906-26913 (2000).

27. C. Schultz. *Bioorg. Med. Chem.* (2003).

28. M. J. Stutts, B. C. Rossier, and R. C. Boucher. Cystic fibrosis transmembrane conductance regulator inverts protein kinase A-mediated regulation of epithelial sodium channel single channel kinetics. *J. Biol. Chem.* **272**, 14037-14040 (1997).

29. J. Konig, R. Schreiber, T. Voelcker, M. Mall, and K. Kunzelmann. The cystic fibrosis transmembrane conductance regulator (CFTR) inhibits ENaC through an increase in the intracellular Cl$^-$ concentration. *EMBO Rep.* **2**, 1047-1051 (2001).

30. T. E. Gray, K. Guzman, C. W. Davis, L. H. Abdullah, and P. Nettesheim. Mucociliary differentiation of serially passaged normal human tracheobronchial epithelial cells. *Am. J. Respir. Cell. Mol. Biol.* **14**, 104-112 (1996).

Chapter 10

VITAMIN C AND FLAVONOIDS POTENTIATE CFTR CL TRANSPORT IN HUMAN AIRWAY EPITHELIA

Horst Fischer and Beate Illek
Children's Hospital Oakland Research Institute (CHORI), 5700 Martin Luther King Jr. Way, Oakland, CA 94609, USA. Telephone (510) 450-7699, fax (510) 450-7910, email: billek@chori.org

1.   INTRODUCTION

A great deal of work has identified the height, viscosity and composition of the airway surface liquid ASL as critical parameters for normal airway function.[1,2] The ionic composition of the ASL is determined by the ion transport mechanisms of the airway epithelium. The cystic fibrosis transmembrane conductance regulator (CFTR), functions as a cAMP-regulated chloride channel, and controls other ion conductive pathways including epithelial chloride and sodium channels. Cystic fibrosis (CF) is caused by defective CFTR function,[3] and is characterized by abnormal sodium and chloride ion transport in several tissues, including the lungs.[4] In the airways obstruction by viscous secretions results in chronic inflammation, with acute exacerbations, followed by secondary bacterial colonization.[5] Interestingly, CF-like symptoms such as thickened airway secretions and bronchiectasis are often seen in patients with airway inflammation. There is emerging evidence that post-translational damage to CFTR by reactive oxygen and nitrogen species decreases CFTR function which may contribute to the development of CF-like symptoms in patients with chronic inflammatory airway diseases without mutations in the CFTR gene.[6] Thus, functional chloride ion transport is a key mechanism for maintaining normal airway functions and healthy lungs.

Over the past years there has been a surge of interest in discovering activators of chloride secretion primarily as drug candidates for CF therapy, but also to increase the hydration of excessive mucus secretions in other inflammatory airway diseases such as asthma, chronic bronchitis and COPD.[7,8] Several candidate molecules have been shown to be effective CFTR activators *in vitro* or *in vivo*.[9] The discovery of small molecules that activate CFTR either directly or through stimulation of CFTR-regulatory pathways will be useful in CF therapy either alone or in combinations with gene therapy. In the past years we have focused on CFTR activators from a list of dietary supplements, which are generally recognized as safe for human health. The flavonoids genistein, apigenin, kaempferol and quercetin effectively activated normal, ΔF508 and G551D mutated CFTR in various tissues and in vivo assays.[10,11] Furthermore there is evidence that genistein interacts directly with the second nucleotide binding domain of CFTR.[12,13]

Vitamin C (L-ascorbate) functions as an important water-soluble antioxidant and is a normal constituent of the ASL.[14,15] Early electrophysiological studies reported a stimulatory effect of ascorbate on Cl transport in frog cornea,[16] and we recently identified CFTR as the underlying target for the activation by vitamin C.[17] The vitamin C content has been quantified from nasal and bronchoalveolar lavages.[14] Assuming that the recovery of airway surface liquid from lavages is approximately 1% of lavage fluid,[18] vitamin C concentrations in the ASL range between 33 to 130 μM in the upper airways and 19 to 49 μM in the lower airways of healthy individuals.[15] A number of conditions are known to severely deplete vitamin C in the ASL or plasma, for example, low levels of ascorbate were found in pediatric and adult patients with bronchial asthma,[19] cystic fibrosis patients,[20,21] in smokers,[22] as well as children exposed to environmental tobacco smoke.[23]

We reasoned that vitamin C may present a safe and cost-effective option for the pharmacological activation of CFTR-mediated chloride ion transport in epithelia. Here we evaluate the efficacy of vitamin C and its epimer D-isoascorbate for the pharmacological stimulation of chloride secretion in normal and CF airways. Furthermore we tested the hypothesis that combined treatment with vitamin C plus flavonoids maximizes epithelial chloride transport.

2.   MATERIALS AND METHODS

Cell culture. The human submucosal serous gland-like cell line Calu-3 was grown in DMEM medium supplemented with 10% fetal calf serum, 4 mM L-glutamine, 100 U/ml penicillin, 100 mg/ml streptomycin. Cystic fibrosis nasal epithelial cells homozygous for ΔF508 CFTR (CF15) were cultured as described.[24,25] Wildtype CFTR-corrected CF15 cells were generated via adenovirus-mediated gene transfer and kindly provided by Dr. T. E. Machen (Department of Molecular and Cell Biology, UC Berkeley). Growth media were nominally free of L-ascorbate (< 10 μM, University Pathology Inc., Salt Lake City, UT). For transepithelial measurements airway epithelial cells were grown to confluency on permeable filter inserts (Falcon, Becton Dickinson, Franklin Lakes, NJ or Snapwell, Corning Costar, Kennebunk, ME) and used after 3 to 10 days.

Short-circuit current measurement. Calu-3 or CF15 epithelial monolayers were mounted into Ussing chambers and short-circuit current was recorded as described.[10] At 20-50 second intervals, transepithelial voltage was clamped to 2 mV for 1 s and the transepithelial resistance (R_{te}) was calculated. A serosa-to-mucosa directed Cl gradient was applied to increase the electrochemical driving force for chloride across the apical membrane. Serosal Ussing chamber solution contained (in mM): 120 NaCl, 20 $NaHCO_3$, 5 $KHCO_3$, 1.2 NaH_2PO_4, 5.6 glucose, 2.5 $CaCl_2$, 1.2 $MgCl_2$. In the mucosal solution, all chloride salts were exchanged for gluconate salts.

Nasal potential difference (NPD) measurements. Measurements of NPD were performed in healthy volunteers as described.[10] Solutions and test drugs were perfused into one nostril at ~5 ml/min at room temperature (23-25°C). NaCl solution contained (in mM): 145 NaCl, 4 KCl, 1 $CaCl_2$, 1 $MgCl_2$, 10 Hepes, pH = 7.4. In Cl free solutions all Cl salts were replaced by the respective gluconate salts. The measured signal was amplified and sampled to a computer.

Cyclic AMP measurements. Confluent Calu-3 cells were incubated with L-ascorbate, D-isoascorbate or forskolin for 15 min and lyzed with 0.1 M HCl. Cellular cAMP levels were measured in non-acetylated samples using a competitive immunoassay for cAMP (R&D systems, Minneapolis, MN).

Drugs and reagents. L-ascorbic acid was made by dissolving the sodium salt of L-ascorbate (tissue culture grade, Sigma) in deionized water. D-isoascorbic acid was dissolved in DMSO. Fresh stock (1 M) and working solutions were prepared daily. Genistein and kaempferol were dissolved as a 10 mM stock solution in DMSO. Forskolin (Calbiochem, La Jolla CA) was dissolved as a 100 mM stock in DMSO and used at 10 μM; isoproterenol was made as a 100 mM stock in water (stored at −20°C) and used at 10 μM; amiloride was made as a 10 mM stock in water and used at 100 μM; N-phenyl anthranilic acid (DPC; Research Biochemicals Inc., Natick MA) was made as 0.5 M stock in ethanol and used at 4 mM; H-89 (N-(2-ethyl)-5-isoquinolinesulfonamide HCl; Calbiochem) was dissolved to 20 mM in DMSO and used at 10 μM; ATP, sodium salt, was prepared as a 100 mM

stock in water and kept frozen at –20°C until use. Chemicals were from
Sigma (St. Louis, MO) if not mentioned otherwise.

3.   RESULTS

Stimulation of chloride secretion by L-ascorbate and D-isoascorbate.
L-ascorbate and D-isoascorbate were effective stimulators of transepithelial
Cl secretion (I_{sc}) across Calu-3 airway epithelia. Figures 1A and 1B show the
dose-dependent stimulation of I_{sc} by L-ascorbate or D-isoascorbate, which
were added to the mucosal and serosal reservoirs of the Ussing chamber. A
maximal dose of L-ascorbate at 1 mM stimulated I_{sc} by 59 ± 20 µA/cm^2 (n =
8) and D-isoascorbate at 300 µM by 37 ± 7 µA/cm^2 (n = 6). The fractional
responses are plotted for each concentration in Fig. 1C and the
corresponding half-maximal stimulatory constants averaged K_m = 80 ± 6 µM
for ascorbate and K_m = 68 ± 10 µM for D-isoascorbate with respective Hill
coefficients of 1.2 ± 0.1 and 1.7 ± 0.3.L-ascorbate and D-isoascorbate were
effective stimulators of transepithelial Cl secretion (I_{sc}) across Calu-3 airway
epithelia. Figures 1A and 1B show the dose-dependent stimulation of I_{sc} by
L-ascorbate or D-isoascorbate, which were added to the mucosal and serosal
reservoirs of the Ussing chamber. A maximal dose of L-ascorbate at 1 mM

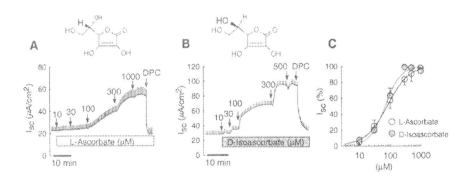

Figure 1. Stimulation of Cl secretion by L-ascorbate and its epimer D-isoascorbate.
Measurement of transepithelial Cl secretion (I_{sc}) across Calu-3 airway epithelia. Time course
of the dose-dependent stimulation of I_{sc} by (A) L-ascorbate (3-oxo-L-gulofuranolactone) and
(B) D-isoascorbate (D-erythro-hex-2-enoic acid γ-lactone). Stimulated Cl currents were
completely inhibited by the Cl channel blocker DPC (4 mM). C. Dose dependency of
ascorbate- and isoascorbate-stimulated Cl currents. Lines are best fits to Michaelis-Menten
kinetics. Half-maximal stimulatory constant averaged 80 ± 6 µM (n = 8) for ascorbate and 68
± 10 µM (n = 6) for D-isoascorbate.

stimulated I_{sc} by 59 ± 20 μA/cm^2 ($n = 8$) and D-isoascorbate at 300 μM by 37 ± 7 μA/cm^2 ($n = 6$). The fractional responses are plotted for each concentration in Fig. 1C and the corresponding half-maximal stimulatory constants averaged $K_m = 80 \pm 6$ μM for ascorbate and $K_m = 68 \pm 10$ μM for D-isoascorbate with respective Hill coefficients of 1.2 ± 0.1 and 1.7 ± 0.3.

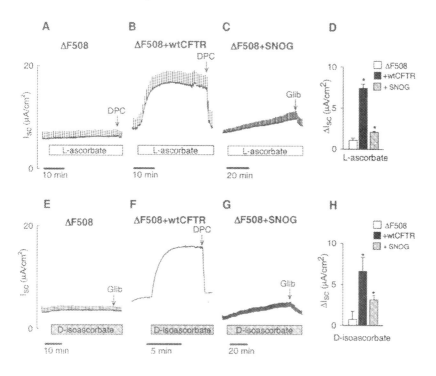

Figure 2. Stimulation of normal and mutant CFTR Cl currents by L-ascorbate and D-isoascorbate. Transepithelial Cl currents (I_{sc}) were measured in nasal CF15 epithelia homozygous for ΔF508 CFTR in the presence of the Na channel blocker amiloride (20 μM). A. L-ascorbate (500 μM, mucosal) failed to stimulate I_{sc} in untreated CF15 epithelia. B. Gene transfer of wildtype CFTR (ΔF508+wtCFTR) recovered the defective Cl secretory response to L-ascorbate. This experiment illustrates that L-ascorbate is specific for the CFTR Cl channel. C. The functional ΔF508 CFTR was determined after correction of the trafficking defect of ΔF508 CFTR using S-nitrosoglutathione (SNOG). SNOG-treated CF 15 epithelia manifested a detectable response to L-ascorbate. D. Summary of ascorbate-stimulated Cl currents. *, Significantly different from ΔF508, P < 0.05; n = 5 - 7 experiments. E. D-isoascorbate (300 μM, mucosal) failed to stimulate I_{sc} in untreated CF15 epithelia. F. Gene transfer of wildtype CFTR (ΔF508+wtCFTR) recovered the defective Cl secretory response to D-isoascorbate. G. SNOG-treated CF15 epithelia manifested a detectable response to D-isoascorbate. D. Summary of isoascorbate-stimulated Cl currents. *, Significantly different from ΔF508, P < 0.05; n = 5 - 7 experiments. Glib, 500 μM glibenclamide.

L-ascorbate and its isomer activate CFTR. We investigated whether the ascorbate- and isoascorbate-stimulated Cl currents were exclusively mediated by the CFTR chloride conductance. This was determined by using the CF15 cell line, which is characterized by the absence of functional CFTR in the apical plasma membrane but the presence of other non-CFTR conductances. We applied one concentration of L-ascorbate (1 mM) or D-isoascorbate (300 µM) that lay within the upper plateau of the dose-response curve and compared L-ascorbate and D-isoascorbate stimulated Cl currents in CF15 vs. wildtype CFTR-corrected CF15 monolayers (Fig. 2). Experiments were performed in the presence of amiloride to block transepithelial Na absorption. In untreated CF15 epithelia, Cl currents were not significantly stimulated by L-ascorbate ($\Delta I_{sc} = 1.1 \pm 0.3$ µA/cm^2, n = 13, Fig. 2A) and D-isoascorbate ($\Delta I_{sc} = 0.7 \pm 1.0$ µA/cm^2, n = 7, Fig. 2E). The defective responses to L-ascorbate and D-Isoascorbate were reversed after gene transfer of wildtype CFTR into CF15 cells such that wtCFTR-corrected CF15 epithelia responded promptly to L-ascorbate ($\Delta I_{sc} = 7.5 \pm 0.5$ µA/cm2, n = 6) or D-isoascorbate ($\Delta I_{sc} = 6.6 \pm 1.7$ µA/cm^2, n = 2). These experiments demonstrated a causal relationship between CFTR expression and the chloride secretory response to either L-ascorbate and D-isoascorbate.

L-ascorbate and D-isoascorbate stimulate ΔF508 CFTR in rescue compound-treated CF airways. Since ascorbates did not activate the trafficking-impaired ΔF508 CFTR (Figs. 2A&H) we investigated whether ΔF508 CFTR could be activated by ascorbates after correction of the trafficking defect using S-nitrosoglutathione (SNOG). SNOG has recently been shown to promote maturation of ΔF508 CFTR protein in both biochemical and functional studies. [26,27]

CF15 monolayers that were treated with 1 mM SNOG for 5 to 24 hours manifested a small but detectable response to L-ascorbate (2.1 ± 0.1, n = 10, L-ascorbate, Fig. 2C) and D-isoascorbate (3.1 ± 0.5, n = 8, D-isoascorbate, Fig. 2G). SNOG treatment recovered the ascorbate and isoascorbate-stimulated Cl secretion between 28 and 47% when compared to using wtCFTR infected CF15 cells (Figs. 2B&F). The summary in Figs. 2D&2G compares the magnitudes of the L-ascorbate and D-isoascorbate stimulated Cl currents in CF15 epithelia. L-ascorbate and D-isoascorbate significantly stimulated chloride currents in both CFTR-infected and SNOG-treated CF15 epithelia.

Roles of protein kinase A and cyclic AMP during ascorbate-stimulated chloride secretion. Protein kinase A is the major kinase that regulates the activity of CFTR. We tested the effect of the protein kinase A inhibitor H-89 on ascorbate (Fig. 3A) and D-isoascorbate (Fig. 3B) stimulated chloride secretion across Calu-3 monolayers in Ussing chambers.

H-89 (10 μM) effectively blocked ascorbate-stimulated (by $56 \pm 5\%$; $n = 3$) and isoascorbate-stimulated Cl secretion (by $20 \pm 6\%$; $n = 3$).

Further, we tested the possibility that ascorbates activated transepithelial Cl secretion via elevation of intracellular cAMP levels. Fig. 3C compares cellular cAMP levels measured in Calu-3 and CF15 cells under resting conditions and after a 15 min exposure to forskolin (10 μM), L-ascorbate (1 mM) or D-isoascorbate (300 μM). Cellular cAMP levels were effectively elevated by the adenylate cyclase activator forskolin in both cell types. In contrast, exposures to L-ascorbate and D-Isoascorbate did not result in a detectable increase of cellular cAMP levels. These data suggest that the activation of CFTR-mediated Cl secretion by L-ascorbate and D-isoascorbate involved a protein kinase A-dependent, but cAMP-independent step.

Ascorbate-stimulated Cl currents are further stimulated by forskolin. We evaluated whether ascorbate shared a common pathway that involved intracellular cAMP signaling. First we determined the effect of the cAMP agonist forskolin on ascorbate-stimulated Cl currents and in a different set of experiments we tested the effect of L-ascorbate on Cl secretion in the presence of forskolin, and thus, elevated cAMP levels. Addition of a maximal dose of L-ascorbate (1 mM, Fig. 4A) stimulated Cl secretion by 44 ± 5 μA/cm^2 in Calu-3 epithelia. Subsequent addition of forskolin further increased Cl secretion to 79 ± 10 μA/cm^2. On average, Cl secretion was stimulated by L-ascorbate to 56% of currents elicited by

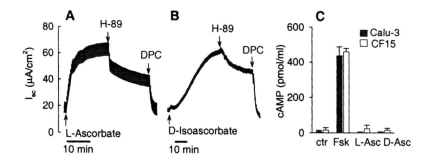

Figure 3. Role of protein kinase A signaling. Addition of the protein kinase A inhibitor H-89 (10 μM) to the mucosal and serosal reservoir of the Ussing chamber partially blocked (A) ascorbate-stimulated and (B) isoascorbate-stimulated Cl currents across Calu-3 airway epithelia. C. Cellular cAMP concentrations in presence of L-ascorbate (L-Asc, 1 mM L-ascorbate) and D-isoascorbate (D-Asc, 300 μM D-isoascorbate) in Calu-3 and CF15 airways. For comparison, resting (ctr) and forskolin-stimulated (Fsk) cAMP levels are shown.

forskolin. In contrast, when the order of drug additions was reversed such that Cl secretion was first stimulated with forskolin, then exposure to L-ascorbate exerted no stimulatory effect on Cl secretion (-1.3 ± 1.0 μA/cm^2, n = 4, not different from zero, one sample t test). The effect of ascorbate on resting and cAMP-stimulated Cl currents is summarized in Fig. 4C. These data indicate that maximally forskolin-activated CFTR is not further

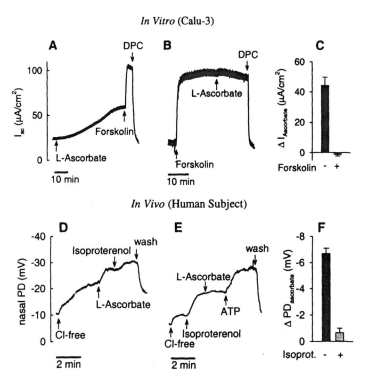

Figure 4. Additivity between L-ascorbate and forskolin in vitro and in vivo. A -C Measurement of transepithelial Cl secretion (I_{sc}) across Calu-3 airway epithelia in vitro. L-ascorbate-stimulated current (1 mM, mucosal) was further increased by forskolin (20 μM, serosal) and completely inhibited by DPC (4 mM). B. In contrast, forskolin-stimulated Cl currents were not further stimulated by L-ascorbate (300 μM, mucosal). C. Summary of ascorbate-stimulated Cl currents in the absence (-) and presence of forskolin (+). D-F. Measurement of nasal potential difference (nasal PD) in a human subject in vivo. D. Perfusion of the nasal floor with L-ascorbate (300 μM) in amiloride-containing Cl free solutions hyperpolarized nasal PD. Response to the β-adrenergic agonist isoproterenol (10 μM) is shown for comparison. Wash, washout with saline. E. In contrast, the isoproterenol-stimulated hyperpolarization of nasal PD was not further activated by L-ascorbate. Note that the calcium-elevating agonist ATP (100 μM) hyperpolarized nasal PD effectively in the presence of isoproterenol and L-ascorbate. F. Summary of ascorbate-induced hyperpolarization of nasal PD in the absence (-) and presence of isoproterenol (Isoprot.) (+).

activated by ascorbic acid suggesting a common signaling pathway for the activation of CFTR by ascorbate and forskolin.

L-ascorbate stimulated chloride transport *in vivo.* The effects of ascorbate were further tested in nasal potential difference (NPD) measurements in healthy volunteers in order to verify the significance of the transepithelial results *in vivo* in humans. Two protocols were used: L-ascorbate was instilled onto the nasal floor either in unstimulated noses or in isoproterenol-stimulated noses. During the initial perfusion with NaCl Ringers the basal NPD = -18.6 ± 1.6 mV ($n = 8$ measurements on 2 subjects). Perfusion with 100 μM amiloride resulted in a depolarization of NPD to -8.5 ± 1.7 mV. The recording in Fig. 4D&E show effects in amiloride-treated noses. Perfusion with Cl free solution (in the continuous presence of amiloride) hyperpolarized NPD by -6.2 ± 1.3 mV ($n = 8$) indicating a Cl-selective, basal conductance in nasal epithelium. Subsequent addition of L-ascorbate hyperpolarized NPD by an additional -6.7 ± 0.4 mV ($n = 3$) which was further hyperpolarized with the cAMP agonist isoproterenol (Fig. 4D).

When NPD was first stimulated with isoproterenol (by -6.5 ± 1.7 mV, $n = 3$) subsequent perfusion with L-ascorbate showed no significant effects (Fig. 4E, -0.8 ± 0.6 mV, not different from zero, one sample t test). However, in the presence of L-ascorbate and isoproterenol, 100 μM ATP hyperpolarized NPD further by -7.4 ± 2.1 mV. These *in vivo* findings were similar to the *in vitro* measurements in Ussing chambers (compare Figs. 4A-C with Figs. 4D-E).

Flavonoids potentiate ascorbate-stimulated chloride currents. Flavonoid compounds are widely used as CFTR openers and we determined a possible interaction between flavonoids and ascorbate during the activation of CFTR. We first chose to investigate the effect of the flavonoid kaempferol, which is both a CFTR opener and a biological antioxidant. In addition, we tested the isoflavone genistein which is a widely used CFTR opener. Fig. 5A illustrates that ascorbate-stimulated Cl currents are additively activated by kaempferol (by 16 ± 2 μA/cm^2, $n = 6$). Reversing the order of the experiment such that L-ascorbate was added to flavonoid-stimulated Cl currents potentiated transepithelial Cl transport as well (by 32 ± 6 μA/cm^2, $n = 5$, Fig. 5C). The addition of the cAMP-agonist forskolin resulted in maximal activation of the ascorbate- and kaempferol-stimulated Cl currents. The fractional responses to ascorbate averaged 42% of the maximal currents evoked in the presence of all three CFTR activators (ascorbate, kaempferol and forskolin), which was increased to 62% by subsequent exposure to kaempferol. These experiments indicated that ascorbate activated CFTR by a different mechanism than the flavonoids kaempferol and genistein.

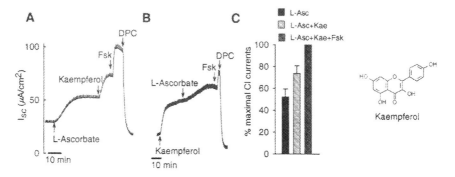

Figure 5. L-ascorbate and the flavonoid kaempferol (3,4',5,7-tetrahydroxyflavone; 3,5,7-trihydroxy-2-(4-hydroxyphenyl)-4H-1-benzopyran-4-one) potentiate CFTR-mediated Cl secretion. Measurement of transepithelial Cl secretion (I_{sc}) across Calu-3 airway epithelia in vitro. A. Effective stimulation of Isc by L-ascorbate (1 mM). The ascorbate-stimulated Cl current was additively increased by kaempferol (20 µM) and forskolin (20 µM). Maximal stimulated Isc by the three CFTR activators was completely blocked by DPC (4 mM, mucosal). B. Effective and sustained stimulation of I_{sc} by kaempferol. The kaempferol-stimulated I_{sc} was stepwise increased by L-ascorbate (3 mM) and forskolin and completely blocked by DPC. C. Fractional I_{sc} responses to L-ascorbate (L-Asc, 1 mM) and to L-ascorbate and kaempferol (L-Asc+Kae). Maximal response to combined stimulation by L-ascorbate, kaempferol, and forskolin. (L-Asc+Kae+Fsk) was defined as 100%.

Similarly genistein (20 µM mucosal) increased ascorbate-stimulated Cl currents across Calu-3 monolayers, by on average 17 ± 4 µA/cm^2 ($n = 3$, Fig. 6A). In monolayers stimulated successively with L-ascorbate and forskolin, genistein further activated I_{sc} by 18 ± 1 µA/cm^2, $n = 9$ (not shown). This effect was also tested in NPD measurements (Fig. 6B). In close agreement with the transepithelial measurements, NPD was progressively hyperpolarized by L-ascorbate (by 6.1 ± 1.1 mV, $n = 2$), genistein (by -7.4 ± 1.4 mV) and isoproterenol (by -5.5 ± 0.5 mV).

4.   DISCUSSION

This study shows that both isoforms of vitamin C, L-ascorbate and D-isoascorbate, effectively activate CFTR-mediated Cl secretion. Their stimulatory effects are potentiated by flavonoids. Trafficking-defective ΔF508 CFTR currents were detectably stimulated by ascorbates after treatment with the SNOG compound, and gene transfer of wildtype CFTR restored the Cl secretory responses to ascorbates indicating the requirement of functional CFTRs for the activation by vitamin C in cystic fibrosis epithelia.

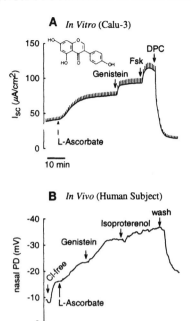

Figure 6. L-ascorbate and the isoflavone genistein (4',5,7-trihydroxyisoflavone; 5,7-dihydroxy-3-(4-hdroxyphenyl)-4H-1-benzopyran-4-one) potentiate CFTR-mediated Cl transport. Measurement of transepithelial Cl secretion (I_{sc}) across Calu-3 airway epithelia in vitro. A. Effective stimulation of I_{sc} by L-ascorbate (1 mM). Ascorbate-stimulated I_{sc} is stepwise increased by genistein (20 µM) and forskolin (20 µM). Maximally stimulated I_{sc} by the three CFTR activators is completely blocked by DPC (4 mM, mucosal). B. Measurement of nasal potential differences (nasal PD) in a human subject in vivo. Perfusion of the nasal floor with L-ascorbate (300 µM) in amiloride-containing chloride free solutions (Cl-free) hyperpolarized nasal PD. The ascorbate-induced hyperpolarization of nasal PD is stepwise increased by genistein and the β-adrenergic agonist isoproterenol (10 µM). Wash, washout with saline.

Vitamin C as a CFTR drug. A surprisingly heterogeneous array of molecules has been found to activate CFTR, such as phenylimidazothiazoles,[28] xanthines,[29-31] phosphatase inhibitors,[32,33] phosphodiesterase inhibitors,[34,35] fluorescein,[36] benzoquinoliziniums,[37,38] or flavonoids.[10-13,39] This range of molecules suggests a number of different drug targets in the regulatory pathway of CFTR. High-throughput assays are likely to add additional compounds to this list.[40] All of the current CFTR activators are useful laboratory tools, however, the use in humans has been hampered by the general non-specificity of the compounds. Although vitamin C is not a specific or drug-like compound, it has the great advantage that it is an essential micronutrient and considered safe for human use. Vitamin C is on the FDA's list of substances that are generally recognized as safe. The upper intake level of vitamin C for humans has been recently set to 2.0 g/day based on its side effect for causing diarrhea in some individuals.[41] The available data from past and current research examining potential adverse effects of supplemental vitamin C indicate that very high intakes of vitamin C (2-4 g/day) are biologically well tolerated.[42]

Maximal effects on CFTR were seen at concentrations of vitamin C at 300 μM (Fig. 1C). However, plasma vitamin C concentrations do not exceed 100 μM even at high oral doses of >1g.[43] Therefore, local delivery of vitamin C to the airway lumen via inhalation may be more advantageous because this route will yield considerably higher concentrations at the target tissue.

Naturally occurring compounds and CFTR. Both flavonoids and vitamin C occur in fruits and vegetables and are present in a healthy diet. Previously we have tested a number of flavonoid compounds of which many showed effects on CFTR activity.[10,44] In this report we selected kaempferol and genistein as two members of naturally occurring flavonoids. We show that the effects of vitamin C and flavonoids were additive, such that a considerable fraction of maximal chloride current was activated by their combined use. The dietary intake of flavonoids results in blood concentrations in the low micromolar concentrations.[45] Acute maximal effects on CFTR currents by single flavonoids were seen at 20 to 40 μM concentrations dependent on the compound.[10] However, owing to the additivity between flavonoids and vitamin C, a dietary effect of these nutraceuticals on the activity of CFTR appears possible. It is noteworthy that a link between fruit consumption and pulmonary function has been found.[46] In particular, vitamin C deprivation has been associated with the risk of asthma.[46] The current recommended dietary allowance for vitamin C is 75 mg. Recently published dietary intake data showed that approximately 25% of the U.S. population did not meet the recommended dietary intake levels for vitamin C. This dietary deficit is reflected in the distribution of vitamin C levels in the population. For example, 50% U.S. females and 75% of U.S. males fall below an optimal blood level of vitamin C, and an alarming 25% of U.S. men aged 31-50 are diagnosed with hypovitaminose C. Serum levels for vitamin C are defined as normal between 29 μM to 90 μM,[43] and a similar range is found in the epithelial lining fluid.[15] Our data suggest that these concentrations will significantly affect the activity of CFTR.

Physiological function of vitamin C in the airways. The function of the airways is to filter particles and bacteria out of the inhaled air and thus keep the lower lungs clean and sterile. This function is performed by the ciliated cells. The composition of the ASL is critical for normal ciliary movement and mucociliary clearance. Salt and water content of the ASL is regulated by epithelial ion transport mechanisms. Normal ASL contains vitamin C. One important function of vitamin C is to protect the airways from oxidative damage by environmental oxidants present in inhaled air.[47] A role for vitamin C in salt and water transport across the airway epithelium has not been considered previously. Dehydration of the mucus lining of the airways results in obstruction of mucociliary clearance leading to airway infections. Our data show that the topical exposure of the nasal mucosa to vitamin C stimulated CFTR-mediated chloride transport into the ASL in a sustained fashion. This data suggests that vitamin C is a determinant for the steady state of salt and water transport in the airways. Thus, we propose that vitamin C supports normal airway function by controlling salt and water secretion by the epithelium. Vitamin C is a novel biological CFTR chloride channel opener and vitamin C alone or in combination with flavonoids may present a novel complementary and alternative medicine approach for the treatment of sticky airway secretions in chronic airway diseases.

ACKNOWLEDGMENT

This study was supported in part by grants from the National Institutes of Health and the Cystic Fibrosis Foundation (Illek02G0).

REFERENCES

1. R. C. Boucher. Regulation of airway surface liquid volume by human airway epithelia. *Pflügers Arch. - Eur. J. Physiol.* **445**, 495-498 (2003).
2. J. H. Widdicombe. Altered NaCl concentration of airway surface liquid in cystic fibrosis. *News in Physiol. Sci.* **14**, 126-127 (1999).
3. J. M. Rommens, M. C. Iannuzzi, B. Kerem, M. L. Drumm, G. Melmer, M. Dean, R. Rozmahel, J. L. Cole, D. Kennedy, and N. Hidaka. Identification of the cystic fibrosis gene: chromosome walking and jumping. *Science* **245**, 1059-1065 (1989).
4. M. J. Welsh and A. E. Smith. Cystic fibrosis. *Scientific American* **273**, 52-59 (1995).
5. P. B. McCray Jr., J. Zabner, H. P. Jia, M. J. Welsh, and P. S. Thorne. Efficient killing of inhaled bacteria in DeltaF508 mice: role of airway surface liquid composition. *Am. J. Physiol. Lung Cell. Mol. Physiol.* **277**, L183-L190 (1999).
6. Z. Bebok, K. Varga, J. K. Hicks, C. J. Venglarik, T. Kovacs, L. Chen, K. M. Hardiman, J. F. Collawn, E. J. Sorscher, and S. Matalon. Reactive oxygen nitrogen species decrease cystic fibrosis transmembrane conductance regulator expression and cAMP-mediated Cl-secretion in airway epithelia. *J. Biol. Chem.* **277**, 43041-43049 (2002).
7. M. R. Knowles and R. C. Boucher. Mucus clearance as a primary innate defense mechanism for mammalian airways. *J. Clin. Invest.* **109**, 571-577 (2002).

8. J. A. Nadel. Role of Neutrophil Elastase in Hypersecretion During COPD Exacerbations, and Proposed Therapies. *Chest* 117, 386-389 (2000).

9. B. Illek, H. Fischer, and T. E. Machen. Genetic disorders of membrane transport. II. Regulation of CFTR by small molecules including HCO3. *Am. J. Physiol. Gastro. and Liver Physiol.* 275, G1221-1226 (1998).

10. B. Illek, B. and H. Fischer. Flavonoids stimulate Cl conductance of human airway epithelium in vitro and in vivo. *Am. J. Physiol. Lung Cell. and Mol. Physiol.* 275, L902-L910 (1998).

11. B. Illek, L. Zhang, N. C. Lewis, R. B. Moss, J.-Y. Dong, and H. Fischer. Defective function of the cystic fibrosis-causing mutation G551D is recovered by genistein. *Am. J. Physiol. Cell Physiol.* 277, C833-C839 (1999).

12. P. J. French, J. Bijman, A. G. Bot, W. E. Boomaars, B. J. Scholte, and H. R. de Jonge. Genistein activates CFTR Cl- channels via a tyrosine kinase- and protein phosphatase-independent mechanism. *Am. J. Physiol. Cell Physiol.* 273, C747-753 (1997).

13. F. Weinreich, P. G. Wood, J. R. Riordan, and G. Nagel. Direct action of genistein on CFTR. *Pflügers Arch.* 434, 484-491 (1997).

14. R. Slade, K. Crissman, J. Norwood, and G. Hatch. Comparison of antioxidant substances in bronchoalveolar lavage cells and fluid from humans, guinea pigs, and rats. *Exp. Lung Res.* 19, 469-484 (1993).

15. A. van der Vliet, C. A. O'Neill, C. E. Cross, J. M. Koostra, W. G. Volz, B. Halliwell, et al. Determination of low-molecular-mass antioxidant concentrations in human respiratory tract lining fluids. *Am. J. Physiol. Lung Cell. Mol. Physiol.* 276, L289-296 (1999).

16. W. N. Scott and D. F. Cooperstein. Ascorbic acid stimulates chloride transport in the amphibian cornea. *Invest. Ophthalmol.* 14, 763-766 (1975).

17. H. Fischer, C. Schwarzer, and B. Illek. Vitamin C controls the CFTR Cl channel. *Proc. Natl. Acad. Sci. U.S.A.* 101, 3692-3696 (2004).

18. S. I. Rennard, G. Basset, D. Lecossier, K. M. O'Donnell, P. Pinkston, P. G. Martin, and R G. Crystal. Estimation of volume of epithelial lining fluid recovered by lavage using urea as marker of dilution. *J. Appl. Physiol.* 60, 532-538 (1986).

19. F. J. Kelly, I. Mudway, A. Blomberg, A. Frew, and T. Sanstorm. Altered lung antioxidant status in patients with mild asthma. *Lancet* 354, 482-483 (1999).

20. R. K. Brown, H. Wyatt, J. F. Price, and F. J. Kelly. Pulmonary dysfunction in cystic fibrosis is associated with oxidative stress. *Eur. Respir. J.* 9(2), 334-339 (1996).

21. B. M. Winklhofer-Roob, H. Ellemunter, M. Fruhwirth, S. E. Schlegel-Haueter, G. Khoschsorur, H. M. A. van't, and D.H. Shmerling. Plasma vitamin C concentrations in patients with cystic fibrosis: evidence of associations with lung inflammation. *Am. J. Clin. Nutr.* 65, 1858-1866 (1997).

22. J. Lykkesfeldt, S. Loft, J. B. Nielsen, and H. E. Poulsen. Ascorbic acid and dehydroascorbic acid as biomarkers of oxidative stress caused by smoking. *Am. J. Clin. Nutr.* 65(4), 959-963 (1997).

23. A. M. Preston, C. Rodriguez, C. E. Rivera, and H. Sahai. Influence of environmental tobacco smoke on vitamin C status in children. *Am. J. Clin. Nutr.* 77, 167-172 (2003).

24. D. M. Jefferson, J. D. Valentich, F. C. Marini, S. A. Grubman, M. C. Iannuzzi, H. L. Dorkin, M. Li, K. W. Klinger, and M. J. Welsh. Expression of normal and cystic fibrosis phenotypes by continuous airway epithelial cell lines. *Am. J. Physiol. Lung Cell. Mol. Physiol.* 259, L496-505 (1990).

25. L. A. Sachs, W. E. Finkbeiner, and J. H. Widdicombe. Effects of media on differentiation of cultured human tracheal epithelium. *In Vitro Cell Dev. Biol. Anim.* 39, 56-62 (2003).

26. M. Howard, H. Fischer, J. Roux, B. C. Santos, S. R. Gullans, P. H. Yancey, and W. J. Welch. Mammalian Osmolytes and S-Nitrosoglutathione Promote ΔF508 Cystic Fibrosis Transmembrane Conductance Regulator (CFTR) Protein Maturation and Function. *J. Biol. Chem.* **278**, 35159-35167 (2003).

27. K. Zaman, M. McPherson, J. Vaughan, J. Hunt, F. Mendes, B. Gaston, and L. A. Palmer. S-nitrosoglutathione increases cystic fibrosis transmembrane regulator maturation. *Biochem. Biophys. Res. Commun.* **284**, 65-70 (2001).

28. F. Becq, B. Verrier, X. B. Chang, J. R. Riordan, and J. W. Hanrahan. cAMP- and Ca^{2+}-independent activation of cystic fibrosis transmembrane conductance regulator by phenylimidazothiazole drugs. *J. Biol. Chem.* **271**, 16171-16179 (1996).

29. V. Chappe, Y. Mettey, J. M. Vierfond, J. W. Hanrahan, M. Gola, B. Verrier, and F. Becq. Structural basis for specificity and potency of xanthine derivatives as activators of the CFTR chloride channel. *Br. J. Pharmacol.* **123**, 683-693 (1998).

30. O. Eidelman, C. Guay-Broder, P. J. van Galen, K. A. Jacobson, C. Fox, R. J. Turner, Z. I. Cabantchik, and H. B. Pollard. A1 adenosine-receptor antagonists activate chloride efflux from cystic fibrosis cells. *Proc. Natl. Acad. Sci. U.S.A.* **89**, 5562-5566 (1992).

31. C. M. Haws, I. B. Nepomuceno, M. E. Krouse, H. Wakelee, T. Law, Y. Xia, H. Nguyen, and J. J. Wine. DF508-CFTR channels: kinetics, activation by forskolin, and potentiation by xanthines. *Am. J. Physiol. Cell Physiol.* **270**, C1544-1555 (1996).

32. F. Becq, T. J. Jensen, X. B. Chang, A. Savoia, J. M. Rommens, L. C. Tsui, M. Buchwald, J. R. Riordan, and J. W. Hanrahan. Phosphatase inhibitors activate normal and defective CFTR chloride channels. *Proc. Natl. Acad. Sci. U.S.A.* **91**, 9160-9164 (1994).

33. H. Fischer, B. Illek, and T. E. Machen. Regulation of CFTR by protein phosphatase 2B and protein kinase C. *Pflügers Arch.* **436**, 175-181 (1998).

34. T. J. Kelley, L. Al-Nakkash, C. U. Cotton, and M. L. Drumm. Activation of endogenous deltaF508 cystic fibrosis transmembrane conductance regulator by phosphodiesterase inhibition. *J. Clin. Invest.* **98**, 513-520 (1996).

35. T. J. Kelley, L. Al-Nakkash, and M. L. Drumm. CFTR-mediated chloride permeability is regulated by type III phosphodiesterases in airway epithelial cells. *Am. J. Resp. Cell Mol. Biol.* **13**, 657-64 (1995).

36. Z. Cai and D. N. Sheppard. Fluorescein derivatives stimulate wild type and mutant CFTR Cl channels (abstract). *Ped. Pulmonol. Suppl.* **20**, 193 (2000).

37. F. Becq, Y. Mettey, M. A. Gray, L. J. Galietta, R. L. Dormer, M. Merten, T. Metaye, V. Chappe, C. Marvingt-Mounir, O. Zegarra-Moran, R. Tarran, L. Bulteau, R. Derand, M. M. Pereira, M. A. McPherson, C. Rogier, M. Joffre, B. E. Argent, D. Sarrouilhe, W. Kammouni, C. Figarella, B. Verrier, M. Gola, and J. M. Vierfond. Development of substituted Benzo[c]quinolizinium compounds as novel activators of the cystic fibrosis chloride channel. *J. Biol. Chem.* **274**, 27415-27425 (1999).

38. R. Derand, L. Bulteau-Pignoux, Y. Mettey, O. Zegarra-Moran, L. D. Howell, C. Randak, L. J. V. Galietta, J. A. Cohn, C. Norez, L. Romio, J.-M. Vierfond, M. Joffre, and F. Becq. Activation of G551D CFTR channel with MPB-91: regulation by ATPase activity and phosphorylation. *Am. J. Physiol. Cell Physiol.* **281**, C1657-1666 (2001).

39. B. Illek, H. Fischer, G. F. Santos, J. H. Widdicombe, T. E. Machen, and W. W. Reenstra. cAMP-independent activation of CFTR Cl channels by the tyrosine kinase inhibitor genistein. *Am. J. Physiol. Cell Physiol.* **268**, C886-893 (1995).

40. L. V. J. Galietta, S. Jayaraman, and A. S. Verkman. Cell-based assay for high-throughput quantitative screening of CFTR chloride transport agonists. *Am. J. Physiol. Cell Physiol.* **281**, C1734-1742 (2001).

41. Food and Nutrition Board Institute of Medicine, Panel on Dietary Antioxidants and Related Compounds, Subcommittees on Upper Reference Levels of Nutrients and Interpretation and Uses of Dietary Reference Intakes, and Standing Committee on the Scientific Evaluation of Dietary Reference Intakes. Dietary Reference Intake. In: Dietary Reference Intakes for Vitamin C, Vitamin E, Selenium, and Carotenoids. (National Academic Press, Washington DC, 2002) pp. 95-185.

42. C. S. Johnston. Biomarkers for establishing a tolerable upper intake level for vitamin C. *Nutr. Rev.* **57**, 71-77 (1999).

43. M. Levine, C. Conry-Cantilena, Y. Wang, R. W. Welch, P.W. Washko, K.R. Dhariwal, J.B. Park, A. Lazarev, J.F. Graumlich, J. King, and L.R. Cantilena. Vitamin C pharmacokinetics in healthy volunteers: Evidence for a recommended dietary allowance. *Proc. Natl. Acad. Sci. U.S.A.* **93**, 3704-3709 (1996).

44. B. Illek, M. E. Lizarzaburu, V. Lee, M. H. Nantz, M. J. Kurth, and H. Fischer. Structural determinants for activation and block of CFTR-mediated chloride currents by apigenin. *Am. J. Physiol. Cell Physiol.* **279**, C1838-1846 (2000).

45. K. Janssen, R. P. Mensink, F. J. Cox, J. L. Harryvan, R. Hovenier, P. C. Hollman, and M. B. Katan. Effects of the flavonoids quercetin and apigenin on homeostasis in healthy volunteers: results from an in vitro and a dietary supplement study. *Am. J. Clin. Nutr.* **67**, 255-262 (1998).

46. J. Schwartz and S. T. Weiss. Relationship between dietary vitamin C intake and pulmonary function in the First National Health and Nutrition Examination Survey (NHANES I). *Am. J. Clin. Nutr.* **59**, 110-114 (1994).

47. R. P. Bowler and J. D. Crapo. Oxidative stress in airways. *Am. J. Resp. Crit. Care Med.* **166**, 538-543 (2002).

Chapter 11

AIRWAY GLYCOCONJUGATES SECRETED IN CYSTIC FIBROSIS AND SEVERE CHRONIC AIRWAY INFLAMMATION RELATIONSHIP WITH *PSEUDOMONAS AERUGINOSA*

Philippe Roussel
Département de Biochimie, Faculté de Médecine & Université de Lille 2, Place de Verdun, 59045 Lille, France.

1. INTRODUCTION

Chronic airway infection by *Pseudomonas aeruginosa* is observed in patients suffering from cystic fibrosis, early in life, and in a few adult patients suffering for chronic bronchitis, after a very long evolution.

Cystic fibrosis (CF) is the most frequent severe genetic disease among Caucasians. In its most typical form, it affects the exocrine glands with the main symptoms being chronic pulmonary disease, pancreatic insufficiency with fat malabsorption, meconium ileus at birth (in 10% CF neonates) and later in life, cirrhosis and male sterility. The hallmark of the disease is an increase of sweat electrolytes (sweat chloride $\geq$ 70 mEq/l).

In cystic fibrosis, there is mucus hypersecretion as in chronic bronchitis. However, unlike most cases of chronic bronchitis, lung infection in CF is unusual and characterized by infection due to *Staphylococcus aureus* or *Haemophilus influenzae* in early life and, rapidly if not directly, by *Pseudomonas aeruginosa*, which is almost impossible to eradicate and is responsible for most of the morbidity and mortality of the disease.[1]

Cystic fibrosis is due to mutations of a gene (*Cftr*) localized on chromosome 7, encoding for a membrane glycoprotein, the CFTR (cystic fibrosis transmembrane conductance regulator).[2] CFTR is a chloride channel of low conductance activated by protein kinase A, which influences other ion channels, such as the sodium channel ENac and the chloride channel ORCC,[3] and which has probably additional unknown functions in cellular physiology which influence this susceptibility to infection.

Nearly 1000 mutations of the CF gene have been observed so far, however, in the American and Northern European populations, one mutation, the deletion of a phenylalanine residue (ΔF508), is found in about 70% of the CF chromosomes and more than 90% of the CF patients have at least one ΔF508 allele.[2] This ΔF508 mutation generates a trafficking defect since most of the mutated CFTR fails to be processed in the ER and is subsequently degraded.[4]

In spite of the discovery of the CF gene in 1989, the pathophysiology of the lung infection is still mysterious and the treatment of the disease, although improving, is largely empirical. The airway mucosa is normally protected by the muco-ciliary system, which is made of a layer of mucus mobilized by cilia beating in the fluid film covering the surface of the airway epithelium. This system acts as an escalator trapping inhaled particles and microorganisms, which are moved up to the pharynx where they are normally swallowed. It normally maintains the bronchial tree in a sterile state.

In CF, the abnormalities of the fluid phase are still a matter of debate. A decrease in the volume of the fluid phase remaining isotonic is the most favored hypothesis.[5] This affects the functioning of the muco-ciliary escalator. However, the question of water and solute modifications as the predominant factor in the genesis of the lung bacterial colonization is also a matter of controversy.

A main problem in understanding the pathophysiology of CF is to relate these abnormalities to lung infection by *P. aeruginosa*. This bacterium, which is harmless in healthy population, becomes pathogenic whenever a breach occurs in the in the local defenses and may have a tendency to live in biofilms. In the typical forms of CF, the airways are inflamed and infected; they are filled with mucus plugs that have entrapped bacteria and leukocytes and which are difficult to eliminate by the muco-ciliary escalator, phagocytosis, or by coughing (*mucoviscidosis*).

Before the discovery of the CF gene, many investigators have been searching for glycosylation abnormalities of the airways that might pave the way of lung colonization.[6,7] However, abnormalities of glycoconjugates in CF seem to differ from one mucosa to another,[8] and from one cell type to another.[9] Alterations of glycoconjugates from CF airway cells in culture have been described, but these differ from those observed in airway mucus.[10,11] Therefore even in a given tissue, i.e. human airways, it seems difficult to explain these various abnormalities by a unique mechanism.

Different types of cells are involved in the airway disease, and not all of these different cells may express CFTR.

In CF patients, airway inflammation, which is characterized by an influx of neutrophils and high levels of proinflammatory cytokines, has been described as early, severe and sustained.[12] It has been suspected that inflammation might occur before bacterial colonization.[13-15] However, recent clinical data suggest that, while a significant relationship between infection and inflammation was observed, the possibility of intrinsic inflammation could not be excluded.[16]

As far as animal models are concerned, the discovery of *cftr* has allowed the development of CF mice, which do not get spontaneously colonized by *Pseudomonas aeruginosa*. However the mice have an airway hyperreactivity.[17,18] Moreover, gene complementation of airway epithelium in the CF mouse is sufficient to correct the inflammatory abnormalities.[19]

The purpose of the present review is to discuss the evidence indicating that there is a relationship between the colonization by *P. aeruginosa* of severely infected airways (mostly in cystic fibrosis) and the modifications of secreted airway glycoconjugates (mucins and proteoglycans).

2.   MUCINS SECRETED BY HUMAN AIRWAYS

Human airway mucins represent a very large family of polydisperse high molecular mass glycoproteins, which are part of the airway innate immunity. In electron microscopy, mucins purified from human bronchial secretion appear as long, polydisperse, linear and apparently flexible threads.[20] Their size varies from a few hundred nanometers up to more than 5 μm, and decreases after reduction of disulfide bridges. They can be schematized as bottle-brush with a peptidic axis, or apomucins, covered by hundreds of carbohydrate chains (Figure 1). Most mucins secreted in the airway lumen are synthesized by the goblet cells and by the mucous cells of the bronchial glands, in contrast to membrane-bound mucins, which are attached to the apical part of other airway epithelial cells.

2.1   Genes encoding airway mucins

Airway apomucins are encoded by, at least, seven different mucin genes, or *MUC*, which are expressed in the airway mucosa.[21-24] MUC1, MUC4, and MUC13 correspond to membrane-bound mucins, whereas MUC2, MUC5B, MUC5AC, MUC19, and MUC7 are secreted in the airway lumen.

O-Glycosylation

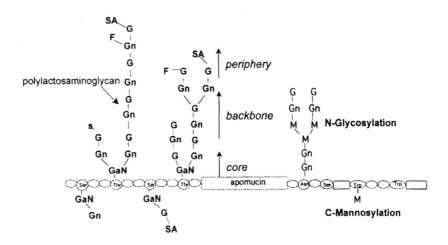

Figure 1. Schematic representation of mucin carbohydrate chains. Most chains are O-glycans, i.e. carbohydrate chains O-glycosidically linked to apomucin by linkages involving N-acetylgalactosamine (GaN) and a hydroxyamino acid (serine or threonine). Each O-glycan can be described with a core, a backbone and a periphery. There are also a few N-glycans having the typical central pentasaccharide, which are N-linked to the asparagine residue of a sequon (Asn-X-Ser [or Thr]), and possibly C-mannosyl residues attached to the tryptophan residue of a sequence (Trp-X-X-Trp).[45] F = fucose; G = galactose; Gn = N-acetylglucosamine; GaN = N-acetylgalactosamine; M = mannose; SA = sialic acid; s = sulfate.

The gel-forming mucins, MUC2, MUC5AC, MUC5B and also MUC19, are synthesized in airway goblet cells and/or mucous cells of the tracheo-bronchial glands. These very large mucins are encoded by four genes having large similarities: *MUC2, MUC5AC, MUC5B* belong to a cluster of genes on chromosome 11 (in p15.5), whereas *MUC19* is located on chromosome 12 (Table 1). They have a central polypeptide region with tandem repeats rich in threonine, serine and proline, which may be interspaced with cysteine-rich domains, a conserved C-terminal domain, and domains homologous to domains of the von Willebrand factor (vWF), which are involved in the dimerization and multimerization of these glycoproteins through disulfide bridges (Figure 2). The tandem repeats are highly glycosylated. Some *MUC* genes are polymorphic and code for variable numbers of tandem repeats (VNTR) (Table 1).

Table 1. MUC genes expressed in human airways

Genes	Chromosome	Mucin localization	aa (n)	repeats	VNTR
MUC1	1q21-24	Membrane-bound epithelial cells		20	+
MUC4	3q29	Membrane-bound epithelial cells	4500-8500	16	+
MUC2	11p15.5	Goblet & mucous cells	5179	23	+
MUC5A,C	11p15.5	Goblet cells	5225	8	+
MUC5B	11p15.5	Mucous & goblet cells in chronic obstructive pulmonary disease	5662	29	
MUC19	12q12	Mucous cells	<7000		
MUC7	4q13-q21	Serous cells	377	23	
MUC13	3q13.3	Trachea			

In the airways, membrane-bound mucins, MUC1 and MUC4, are mostly synthesized by non-glandular cells of the epithelium. They have a small cytoplasmic domain, a transmembrane domain, and a large domain stretching out from the epithelium, which is highly glycosylated, and which probably corresponds to the glycocalyx covering these cells. Although parts of these membrane bound-mucins may be shed from the airway mucosa to a certain extent, they cannot be considered as secreted mucins and do not represent a major part of the airway mucus.

2.2   Regulation of *MUC* genes of secreted mucins

The large secreted mucins are synthesized in goblet cells and mucous cells, which express very little CFTR, if any,[25-27] suggesting that, in CF, mucin alterations should occur through a secondary mechanism.

Chen et al[28] have shown that *MUC5B*, which is normally expressed in submucosal mucous cells, could be also expressed in the surface goblet cells of tissue obtained from patients with chronic obstructive pulmonary disease or asthma (Table 1). Goblet cell metaplasia has also been linked to the increase of mucin gene expression.[29]

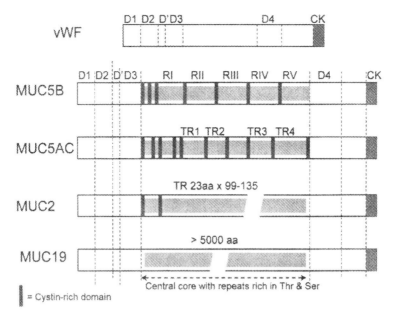

Figure 2. Schematic representation of the organization of apomucins expressed in the airways. Secreted airway mucins have different domains analogous to the von Willebrand factor (vWF): a cystein knot (CK) at their C-terminal end and five domains (D1, D2, D', D3 and D5), which are involved in the dimerization and multimerization of the mucins. The central core, which corresponds to a highly glycosylated domain contain the tandem repeats (TR) sometimes interspaced with cystein-rich domains.

Several inflammatory cytokines, TNFα, IL-1β, IL-4, IL-6, IL-9, IL-13 and IL-17 have been linked to increased mucin gene expression in the airway epithelium (Table 2). Most of these studies were based on undifferentiated or cancerous cell lines and one should probably be careful in extrapolating all these data to in vivo situations. For instance, using an transformed respiratory cell line (MM39), Delmotte *et al*[30] found that it expressed *MUC1* and *MUC4* and that, in certain conditions these cells could express mucin genes (*MUC6*), which are not normally expressed in the human airway mucosa. Moreover, the secreted mucin-like molecules had a much lower molecular mass than the mucins secreted in vivo.

Recently, Chen *et al*[31] have compared the effects of a panel of cytokines (IL-1α, 1β, 2, 3, 4, 5, 6, 7, 8, 9, 10, 11, 12, 13, 15, 16, 17 18 and TNFα) on highly differentiated cultures of primary human tracheo-bronchial epithelial cells and found that the best stimulants for the expression of *MUC5B* and *MUC5AC* were IL-6 and IL-17. They also showed that those cytokines mediated *MUC5B* expression through the ERK signaling pathway and that the IL-17 effect was at least partly mediated through IL-6 by a JAK2-dependent autocrine/paracrine loop.

Table 2. Regulation of mucin genes by cytokines.

Cytokine	Cell type / animal	MUC2	MUC5AC	MUC5B	Ref.
TNFα	NCI-H292	+			32,33
	LS174T	+			34
IL-1β	NCI-H292	+	+		35
IL-4	Transgenic over-expression of IL-4 in mice		+		36
IL-4	NCI-H292	+			37
	LS174T	+			34
IL-6	Primary cells		++	++	31
IL-9	Undifferentiated tracheo-bronchial cells.		+		38
					39
	C7B16 mice		+		40
IL-13	LS174T	+			34
IL-17	Primary cells		++	++	31
EGF,TGFα	NCI-H292				41
LPS	NCI-H292 explants	+	+		42
LTA	HMC3MUC2	+	+		42

The expression of some of mucin genes (at least *MUC2* and *MUC5AC*) is also induced by bacterial products (lipopolysaccharide and flagellin of *Pseudomonas aeruginosa*, lipoteichoic acid of Gram-positive bacteria),[42] as well as by tobacco smoke.[43] Prostaglandin E2 also induces the expression of *MUC5AC*.[33]

There is no indication concerning the regulation of *MUC7* in the airway cells. However, McPherson *et al*[44] have observed a defect in β-adrenergic stimulation of mucin and serous proteins in CF submandibular glands, that could be corrected by compounds related to IBMX. Considering that submandibular glands contain many serous cells expressing CFTR and *MUC7*, one may speculate on the direct role of CFTR on the regulation of *MUC7*.

2.3   Post-translational modifications of mucins

Human airway mucins are highly glycosylated (70-80% per weight). They contain from one single to several hundreds carbohydrate chains. The carbohydrate chains that cover the apomucins are extremely diverse, adding to the complexity of these molecules (Figure 1). So far most of the structural information concerning airway secreted mucins has been obtained for large secreted mucins.

In the RER of goblet cells, few N-glycans are transferred from lipid intermediates to specific asparaginyl residues of apomucin, corresponding to sequons (Asn-X-Ser/or Thr). Recently, Perez-Vilar *et al*[45] have shown that C-mannosylation occurs on specific sequences (Try-X-X-Try) of MUC5B and MUC5AC, likely in the RER, and that this process provided contact regions where mucin oligomers/multimers interact with one another.

However, the vast majority of carbohydrate chains of large secreted mucins are O-glycans. Structural information is available for more than 150 different O-glycan chains corresponding to the shortest chains (less than 12 sugars).[20]

The biosynthesis of these carbohydrate chains is a stepwise process involving many glycosyl- or sulfo-transferases.[20] The only structural element shared by all mucin O-glycan chains is a GalNAc residue linked to a serine or threonine residue of the apomucin (Figure 1). There is growing evidence that the apomucin sequences influence the first glycosylation reactions (initiation of the chains)(reviewed in ref. 20). The elongation of the chains leads to various linear or branched extensions organized as building blocks made of a disaccharide Galβ1-4GlcNAc- (type 2 disaccharide). Some linear chains correspond to lactosaminoglycans.[46] Their non-reducing end, which corresponds to the termination of the chains, may bear different carbohydrate structures corresponding to derivatives of type 1 (Galβ1-3GlcNAc-) or type 2 disaccharides, such as histo-blood groups A or B determinants, H and sulfated H determinants, Lewis a, Lewis b or Lewis y epitopes, as well as sialyl- or sulfo- (sometimes sialyl- and sulfo-) Lewis a or Lewis x determinants.

The synthesis of these different terminal determinants involves different pathways with a whole set of glycosyl- and sulfo-transferases.[20] Figure 3 represents biosynthetic pathways leading to some very common glycotopes derived from type 2 disaccharide unit, such as the H determinant, which is a signature of the Secretor status of an individual, the sulfated or sialylated derivatives of a terminal type 2 disaccharide Galβ1-4GlcNAc, or the various sialylated or/and sulfated derivatives of the Lewis x epitope.

So far most of the structural information concerning the O-glycosylation process has been obtained from bulks of secreted mucins. It is quite possible that the peptide sequence of the different mucins, MUC2, MUC5B, MUC5AC, and MUC19 influence the glycosylation of the different mucins, and the glycosylation of a given apomucin might vary to generate different glycoforms.[47]

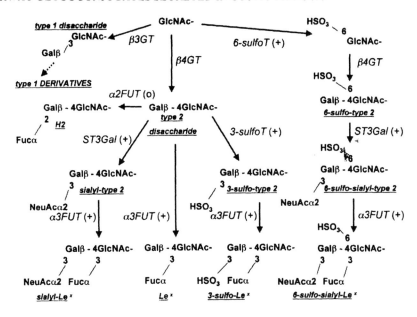

Figure 3. Transferases involved in the biosynthesis of common non-reducing ends of airway mucin O-glycans. ß4GT = UDP-Gal:GlcNAcß1,4-Gal transferase; Gß3 = UDP-Gal:GlcNAcß1,3-Gal transferase; 3-sulfo-T = galactosyl 3-O-sulfotransferase; 6-sulfo-T = N-acetylglucosaminyl-6-O-sulforansferase; α2FUT = α1-2 fucosyltransferase; α3FUT = α1-3 fucosyltransferase;   ST3Gal = α2-3 sialyltransferase, (+) indicates the stimulation of a transferase by TNFα.

Finally, due to their wide structural diversity forming a combinatory of carbohydrate determinants as well as to their location at the surface of the airways, mucins are involved in multiple interactions with microorganisms and are very important in the protection of the underlying airway mucosa.[20]

2.4   Influence of inflammation on the composition of secreted airway mucins

Inflammation as such may modify the synthesis and glycosylation of serum glycoproteins. The increased secretion of acute phase glycoproteins synthesized in the liver in relation to inflammation is well known, but several recent reports have indicated possible glycosylation modifications of acute phase glycoproteins such as an increased expression of sialyl-Lewis x epitopes due to the secretion of cytokines.[48]

In order to determine the influence of chronic and severe inflammation on the post-translational modifications of mucins, Davril *et al*[49] have purified airway mucins from 39 patients suffering either from cystic fibrosis or from chronic bronchitis. The bulk of mucins of each patient was purified using 2 steps of density gradient ultracentrifugation. For each patient, the importance of infection in the mucus secretion was estimated by measuring an index corresponding to the ratio of DNA present in the secretion to the carbohydrate content corresponding to the mucins.

Measuring this index allowed the separation of mucins into four groups: mucins from patients suffering from cystic fibrosis and patients suffering from chronic bronchitis, with or without severe infection. The 39 airway mucin samples were compared for their sialic acid and sulfate contents, as well as for the sialyl-Lewis x expression (Table 3 and 4).

Comparing a group of mucins from CF patients with mucins from other patients, there was a significant increase in the sulfate content of the CF mucins (Table 3). This confirmed previous work showing hypersulfation of glycoproteins or mucins secreted by CF patients).[6,50-53] However, when comparing the mucins from infected patients (CF and non-CF) with those from non-infected patients, the difference was even more significant raising the question of a possible influence of severe inflammation on the sulfation process of airway mucins (Table 3).

The sialic acid content of airway mucins from CF patients and from patients suffering from chronic bronchitis with severe infection was higher than that from non infected patients (Table 4). This was also true for the sialyl-Lewis x reactivity of these different groups of mucins (Table 4).

Table 3. Comparison of the sulfate content of airway mucins secreted by different groups of patients.[49] (* Sulfate is expressed in % by weight)

	Cystic fibrosis (CF) (n = 14)	Chronic bronchitis (CB) (n = 24)	p
Sulfate *	3.31 ± 0.25	2.67 ± 0.56	0.024
	Infected patients (CF + CB) (n=20)	Non-infected patients (CF + CB) (n=18)	
Sulfate	3.16 ± 0.18	2.62 ± 0.15	0.014

Table 4. Sialic acid content and sialyl-Lewis x reactivity of airway mucins secreted by different groups of patients.[49]

	Infected CF (n = 13)	Infected CB (n = 7)	p
Sialic acid *	7.66 ± 0.47	6.30 ± 0.97	NS
Sialyl-Lewis x**	1.19 ± 0.12	1.11 ± 0.09	NS
	Infected patients (CF + CB) (n=20)	Non-infected patients (CF + CB) (n=18)	
Sialic acid	7.18 ± 0.46	3.92 ± 0.41	0.0001
Sialyl-Lewis x	1.16 ± 0.08	0.80 ± 0.11	0.035

* Sialic acid is expressed in N-acetylneuraminic acid % by weight
** The reactivity of the mucin samples with an anti-sialyl-Lewis x antibody was determined in ELISA assay by measuring the absorbance at 490 nm.[49]

Similar modifications of the sialic acid content have been observed in the bulk of salivary mucins secreted by patients suffering from cystic fibrosis. Carnoy et al[54] have shown an increased sialylation of CF salivary mucins as compared to the mucins from controls, and more recently, Shori et al[55] have observed an increased expression of sialyl Lewis x determinants in CF salivary mucins. One should also mention that these data are in agreement with structural studies carried out on the acidic carbohydrate chains of the mucins from a patient suffering from cystic fibrosis severely infected by *Pseudomonas aeruginosa*[56] and from two adult patients suffering from chronic bronchitis without severe infection by *Pseudomonas aeruginosa*.[57,58] Many oligosaccharide bearing sialyl-Lewis x epitopes were observed in the mucins from the CF patient, in contrast to the mucins from the patients suffering from chronic bronchitis without severe infection. Moreover, a recent study of the polylactosaminoglycan chains of the mucins from patients suffering from cystic fibrosis and from chronic bronchitis, with or without severe infection, has shown that mucins from severely infected patients contain more polylactosaminoglycan chains terminated with a sialyl-N-acetyllactosamine group or with a sialyl-Lewis x epitope than the mucins from non-severely infected patients.[46]

2.5 Influence of inflammation on the glycosyl- and sulfo-transferases involved in the biosynthesis of secreted airway mucins

The different modifications observed in the mucins of severely infected patients suffering from cystic fibrosis or from chronic bronchitis strongly suggest that inflammation affects glycosylation and sulfation processes in the airway mucosae of these patients.

TNFα is an important factor of airway mucosa inflammation, acting as an initial inflammatory cytokine that subsequently regulates both early neutrophil infiltration and eosinophil recruitment into the lung and airspace.[59] TNFα, as other cytokines, is found in the airways of patients suffering from bronchial diseases such as chronic bronchitis or cystic fibrosis.[60,61] In order to investigate the role of cytokines on mucin sulfation and glycosylation, explants of human airway mucosa have been exposed to TNFα.[62] The activities of galactosyl 3-O- and N-acetylglucosaminyl-6-O-sulfotransferases, of α1-3 fucosyltransferases and α2-3 sialyltransferases were increased in contrast to that of α1-2 fucosyltransferase, which was not modified (Figure 3).

TNFα also increases messenger expression of α2,3-sialyltransferases *ST3-GalIII* and *ST3-GalIV,* and of α1,3-fucosyltransferases *FUT3* and *FUT4*.[62]

Therefore by acting on these different enzymes, TNFα is involved in the biosynthesis of Lewis x, sialyl-Lewis x, sulfo-Lewis x and sulfo-sialyl-Lewis x determinants by the human bronchial mucosa (Figure 3). In the future, it would be important to find out if other cytokines, which are abundant in CF airways from severely infected patients, influence the glycosylation and/or sulfation of airway mucins and also induce the expression of these particular glycotopes.

CFTR is highly expressed in non-ciliated epithelial cells, in some duct cells and in serous cells of the tubular glands.[25,26] In contrast, the expression of CFTR in cells synthesizing mucins (goblet cells and mucous glands of the acinar cells) is very low, if any.[27] Therefore the effect of the CFTR defect on mucin glycosylation may not be primary but secondary.

2.6 Can the discrepancies in glycosylation between mucins secreted by CF patients and the glycoconjugates synthesized by CF airway cell cultures be explained?

Various abnormalities of glycoconjugates synthesized by CF cells in culture have been described.[10] They usually differ from those observed in secreted mucins.

As mentioned, since airway cells in culture express CFTR (wild type or mutant in CF cells), they probably have a serous, or surface epithelial, rather than a mucous phenotype. In vivo the serous cells secrete glycoproteins, such as bronchotransferrin, which are mostly N-glycosylated, and are therefore very different from mucins secreted by mucous or goblet cells. There are also differences in the sialylation processes between the mucins of the goblet cells (mostly α2-3) and the glycoproteins of the other epithelial cells of the surface (mostly α2-6).[63] However, in most studies performed on airway cells in culture, the glycoproteins that were analyzed, membrane glycoproteins and/or secreted glycoproteins, were not well identified and did not have the typical features of large secreted mucins.

In contrast to what is observed in mucins secreted by CF patients, decreased sialylation of glycoproteins from CF cells has been reported in various CF cells derived from the respiratory mucosa from CF patients).[64,65] Increased fucosylation of glycoconjugates has been observed in CF cells in culture that was reversible when these cells were transfected with wild type cftr.[10,66] The undersialylation was also reversible when these cells were transfected with wild type cftr.

However, in a study using CHO or BHK cells transfected with ΔF508 or wt CF gene, Brockhausen et al[9] showed that several glycosyl- or sulfo-transferases involved in the biosynthesis of mucin type-O glycans by these cells were not modified by transfection with ΔF508 or wt CF gene. As far as sulfation is concerned, the glycoconjugates from CF cells in culture are hypersulfated.[52,67,68] Several hypotheses have been postulated to explain these abnormalities. It has been suggested that, in CF cells, defective acidification of the trans-Golgi network may modify the activity[69] or the cellular localization[66] of several transferases.

However this issue of defective acidification of the *trans*-Golgi network is controversial[70] and it has been recently suggested that there was no defect in acidification but rather a hyperacidification of endosomal organelles in CF lung epithelial cells.[71] It has also been suggested that the concentration of PAPS, the sulfate donor, is regulated in part by CFTR[72] and therefore may influence the sulfation process. The wild-type CFTR would tend to lower the PAPS concentration in the Golgi lumen by letting PAPS leak out of the Golgi, whereas the lack of normal CFTR in CF would increase PAPS concentration in the Golgi and therefore favor sulfation reactions.

Cell lines are indispensable tools in deciphering pathophysiological mechanisms but their phenotype (expression of various glycoprotein genes such as mucin genes, glycosyltransferases, and receptors) may be different from that of the airway cells in their in-vivo environment. In most of the previous studies, the precise phenotype (serous, mucous, non glandular) of the airway cells in culture has not been defined and their ability to express the genes coding for secreted mucins has not been examined. However, since they express CFTR, one might suspect that they do not express these mucin genes.

Few studies have also concerned modifications of glycolipids, especially an increase in asialo-GM1. In vivo, this glycolipid is only expressed on the surface of regenerating cells.[73] It has been observed on the surface of some epithelial cells in primary culture, in a higher percentage of CF respiratory (12 %) than in control cells (2.9 %).[74]

The glycosylation abnormalities observed in glycoconjugates synthesized by serous, mucous, and non-glandular cells might therefore obey to different mechanisms, directly related to CFTR when cells express CFTR, but indirectly when cells do not express CFTR. Finally, the differences in the glycosylation and sulfation between secreted mucins and glycoconjugates synthesized by airway cells in culture strongly suggest that two different types of alterations are observed in the CF airway mucosa:

1. An abnormality of some epithelial cells of the surface, which express mutant CFTR and which involve membrane glycoproteins and glycolipids and is directly related to the CFTR abnormality by an unknown mechanism.

2. Another one in the goblet cells and mucous cells, which do not express CFTR, involves the secreted mucins, the glycosylation of these CF airway mucin producing cells being probably dependent on the action of various mediators such as cytokines.

2.7   Inflammation may favor interactions with *P. aeruginosa*

Pseudomonas aeruginosa is an opportunistic bacterium with a strong tropism for airways of patients suffering from a defect in host defense mechanism. It is responsible for the early colonization of most patients suffering from cystic fibrosis and of a few cases of chronic bronchial diseases, but after a much longer evolution. It can be trapped by mucus of patients suffering from cystic fibrosis and chronic bronchitis, and its niche is constituted by the mucus layer covering the airways.

In CF patients, the vast majority of the *Pseudomonas* cells are mixed with mucins in the airway lumen.[75,76] They bind poorly to intact tracheal cells but bind to injured[77] and regenerating respiratory epithelial cells, which express asialo-GM1.[73] The pilus adhesin of *P. aeruginosa* PAK and PAO bind to asialo-gangliosides, asialo-GM1 and -GM2.[78] The carbohydrate sequence β-D-GalNAc(1->4)β-D-Gal of these asialo-gangliosides is the minimal carbohydrate receptor sequence   for the pilus adhesin of *P. aeruginosa* PAK and PAO.[79] However asialo-GM1 is absent or scarce on the airway epithelium, except for on regenerating cells, thus the role of the bacteria adhering to airway epithelial cells may not be the main factor for the persistent colonization of the CF airways by *P. aeruginosa*.

Pseudomonas aeruginosa recognizes mucins, the main component of mucus and early studies have demonstrated that sialic acid and N-acetylglucosamine were involved in the interactions between *Pseudomonas aeruginosa* and mucins.[80] Airway mucins and salivary mucins from CF patients have been found to have an increased affinity for *Pseudomonas aeruginosa*,[54,81] but all airway mucins studied so far more or less bind this microorganism. It was therefore suggested that *Pseudomonas aeruginosa* had one or several adhesins with affinity for some of the diverse carbohydrate chains covering the airway mucins.[82]

Pseudomonas aeruginosa is a piliated microorganism and pilin has been found to bind to the Galβ1-4GalNAc sequence observed in asialo-GM1. This disaccharide sequence, which is characteristic of gangliosides, has never been found in airway mucins, and, in vivo, should not be an important ligand except on regenerating cells or injured cells.[73]

However the preparation of non-piliated strains of *P. aeruginosa* showed that the bacteria still adhere to mucins, even more strongly,[83] as well as to different glycopeptides obtained by proteolysis of airway mucins.[84] Non-pilus adhesins have been identified using mutated strains of *Pseudomonas aeruginosa* (PAK and PAO1).[82] The observation that non-motile mutants had a low affinity for airway mucins, indicated that proteins of the flagella might be involved in the binding to mucins and the flagellar cap protein (Fli D) of strain PAK has been identified as a major factor of the binding to mucins.[85] More recently the flagellar cap protein (Fli D) and the flagellin (Fli C), of strain PAO1, have been found to be involved in the binding to airway mucins.[86]

In order to identify some of the carbohydrate ligands involved in the binding to *P. aeruginosa*, various approaches have been used. They were mainly based on the use of a single type of oligosaccharide representing the non-reducing end of one of the multiple chains covering the airway mucins.[87-90] These oligosaccharides were either substituted with an hydrophobic tail in order to allow their binding to plastic, or they were hooked to a polyacrylamide to generate a neoglycoconjugate with several identical chains, which, moreover, could be labeled with fluorescein. The binding of these different neoglycoconjugates to various strains of bacteria has been studied using either a microtiter plate adhesion assay or flow cytometry, and various carbohydrate ligands have been defined (Table 5).

The best ligands are the sialyl-Lewis x and the 3-sialyl-6-sulfo-Lewis x determinants.[89,90] Moreover, in the case of the PAO1 strain, specific ligands of the flagellar proteins have been identified, sialyl-Lewis x and Lewis x for the flagellar cap protein, and Lewis x for the flagellin.[86] These ligands were not the specific ligands of the corresponding proteins of the PAK strain.

Table 5. Carbohydrate ligands of *P. aeruginosa* strains

Carbohydrate ligands	*P. aeruginosa* strains	Ref.
Galβ1,4GlcNAcβ1,3Galβ1,4Glc-	M35 (mucoid),	87
	1244 (piliated & non-piliated),	88
	PAK(piliated & non-piliated)	87
Galβ1,3GlcNAcβ1,3Galβ1,4Glc-	M35 (mucoid),	87
	1244 (piliated & non-piliated)	87,88
NeuAcα2,3Galβ1,3GlcNAcβ1,3Gal–	1244 (piliated)	87
Galβ1,3[Fucα1,4]GlcNAc– [*Lewis a*]	1244 (non-piliated) clinical strains	87
Galβ1,4[Fucα1,3]GlcNAc– [*Lewis x*]	1244 (non-piliated) clinical strains	89
Fucα1,2Galβ1,4[Fucα1,3]GlcNAc– [*Lewis y*]	1244 (non-piliated) clinical strains	89
NeuAcα2,3Galβ1,4[Fucα1,3]GlcNAc– [*sialyl-Lewis x*]	1244 (non-piliated) clinical strains	89

Carbohydrate ligands	P. aeruginosa strains	Ref.
3-Sulfo-Galβ1,4[Fucα1,3]GlcNAc– [3-sulfo-Lewiş x]	1244 (non-piliated) clinical strains	89
NeuAcα2,3Galβ1,4[6-sulfo][Fucα1,3] Glc-NAc– [3-sialyl-6-sulfo-Lewiş x]	1244 (non-piliated) clinical strains	90

Neoglycoconjugates are very useful to analyze the affinity of a bacterium for a given type of ligand but it should be noted (i) that they may not reproduce the environment of that ligand in the airway mucin molecule, and (ii) that the affinity of a bacterium for a specific ligand on a mucin molecule or on a neoglycoconjugate may not be necessarily identical.

In summary, the binding of *P. aeruginosa* to airway mucins may involves different carbohydrate ligands, especially the acidic derivatives of the Lewis x determinants induced by inflammation, in cystic fibrosis and in rare cases of chronic bronchitis with a long evolution.

3.   AIRWAY MUCUS PROTEOGLYCANS AND INFECTION

In order to identify alginate in the sputum of patients suffering from cystic fibrosis, Rahmoune *et al*[91] developed a procedure to characterize the different acidic components observed in proteolyzed sputum and to identify alginate among mucin glycopeptides, nucleic acids and glycosaminoglycans. The procedure was based upon agarose electrophoresis and staining with toluidine blue, before or after the action of nucleases and or chondroitinases. It was applied to the sputum of 24 patients suffering either from cystic fibrosis or from chronic bronchitis with or without severe infection. There was very little, if any, alginate in the soluble airway macromolecules from severely infected CF patients; less than 1%. However, Rahmoune *et al*[91] identified chondroitin sulfate in the sputum of all CF patients severely infected by *Pseudomonas aeruginosa*, as well as in the sputum from one patient with chronic bronchitis, whereas CF patients with mild infection had very little chondroitin sulfate. They suggested that the presence of chondroitin sulfate proteoglycans in sputum was not related to CF but to the severity of infection.

These data have been recently confirmed by Khatri *et al*[92] who observed that chondroitinase ABC caused an increased solubility and a 70-90% reduction in turbidity in purulent sputa from CF or non-CF patients, suggesting that the degradation of proteoglycans in purulent mucus might improve airway clearance in chronic respiratory infections.

The chondroitin sulfate containing proteoglycan may correspond at least to proteoglycans secreted by serous cells, especially to decorin,[93] a major product of these cells, although the presence other proteoglycans such as inter-alpha-trypsin inhibitor cannot be eliminated.[94]

It is therefore possible that the secretion of chondroitin sulfate proteoglycan is a marker of severe inflammation acting on serous cells.

4. CONCLUSION

Severe airway inflammation and infection are characterized (i) by increased synthesis and secretion of airway mucins with modifications of their glycosylation and sulfation pattern, and (ii) by secretion of chondroitin sulfate proteoglycan, reflecting the stimulation of the different glandular cells in the airways. The modifications of airway mucins induced by inflammation create different carbohydrate epitopes with a strong affinity for *Pseudomonas aeruginosa,* and most probably play an important role in the chronic airway colonization of CF patients.

Whether or not the severe inflammation in CF is primitive or secondary is another question, and if primary,[95] what is the link between the CFTR defect and inflammation?

ACKNOWLEDGMENTS

I am pleased to acknowledge the long-term collaboration and the fruitful discussions with Dr. Reuben Ramphal from the University of Florida (Gainesville).

REFERENCES

1. M.J. Welsh, L.-C. Tsui, T.F. Boat, and A.L. Beaudet. Cystic fibrosis, in: *The metabolic and molecular bases of inherited disease*, edited by C.R. Scriver, A.L. Beaudet, W.S. Sly, and D. Valle (McGraw-Hill Inc., 1995), pp. 3799-3876.
2. J. Zielenski and L.-C. Tsui. Cystic fibrosis: genotypic and phenotypic variations, *Annu. Rev. Genet.* **29**, 777-807 (1995).
3. S. Devidas and W.B. Guggino. CFTR: domains, structure, and function. *Bioenerg. Biomembr.* **29**, 443-451 (1997).
4. J.R. Riordan. Cystic fibrosis as a disease of misprocessing of the cystic fibrosis transmembrane conductance regulator glycoprotein, *Am. J. Hum. Genet.* **64**, 1499-1504 (1999).

5. H. Matsui, C.W. Davis, R. Tarran, and R.C. Boucher. Osmotic water permeabilities of cultured, well-differentiated normal and cystic fibrosis airway epithelia. *J. Clin. Invest.* **105**, 1418-1427 (2000).

6. P. Roussel, G. Lamblin, P. Degand, E. Walker-Nasir, and R.W. Jeanloz. Heterogeneity of the carbohydrate chains of sulfated bronchial glycoproteins isolated from a patient suffering from cystic fibrosis. *J. Biol. Chem.* **250**, 2114-2122 (1975).

7. T.F. Boat, P.W. Cheng, R. Iyer, D.M. Carlson, and I. Polony. Human respiratory tract secretions. Mucous glycoproteins of nonpurulent tracheobronchioal secretions and sputum of patients with bronchitis and cystic fibrosis. *Arch. Biochem. Biophys.* **117**, 97-104 (1976)

8. T.F. Scanlin and M.C. Glick. Terminal glycosylation in cystic fibrosis. *Biochim. Biophys. Acta* **1455**, 241-253 (1999).

9. I. Brockhausen, F. Vavasseur, and X. Yang. Biosynthesis of mucin type O-glycans: lack of correlation between glycosyltransferase and sulfotransferase activities and CFTR expression. *Glycoconj. J.* **18**, 685-697 (2001).

10. A.D. Rhim, L. Stoykova, M.C. Glick, and T.F. Scanlin. Terminal glycosylation in cystic fibrosis (CF): a review emphasizing the airway epithelial cell. *Glycoconj. J.* **8**, 649-659 (2001).

11. P. Roussel. Airway glycoconjugates and cystic fibrosis. *Glycoconj. J.* **18**, 645-647 (2001).

12. A. Cantin. Cystic fibrosis lung inflammation: early, sustained, and severe. *Am. J. Respir. Crit. Care Med.* **151**, 939-941 (1995).

13. M.W. Konstan, K.A. Hilliard, T.M. Norvell, and M. Berger. Bronchoalveolar lavage findings in cystic fibrosis patients with stable, clinically mild lung diseases suggest ongoing infection and inflammation. *Am. J. Respir. Crit. Care Med.* **150**, 448-454 (1994).

14. T.L. Bonfield, J.R. Panuska, M.W. Konstan, K.A. Hilliard, J.B. Hilliard, H. Ghnaim, and M. Berger. Inflammatory cytokines in cystic fibrosis lungs. *Am. J. Respir. Crit. Care Med.* **152**, 2111-2118 (1995).

15. J.F. Chmiel, M. Berger, and M.W. Konstan. The role of inflammation in the pathophysiology of CF lung disease. *Clin. Rev. Allergy Immunol.* **23**, 5-27 (2002).

16. J.C. Dakin, A.H. Numa, H. Wang., J.R. Morton, C.C. Vertzyas, and R.L. Henry. Inflammation, infection, and pulmonary function in infants and young children with cystic fibrosis. *Am. J. Respir. Crit. Care Med.* **165**, 904-910 (2002).

17. A. van Heeckeren, R. Walenga, M.W. Konstan, T. Bonfield, P.B. Davis, and T. Ferkol. Excessive inflammatory response of cystic fibrosis mice to bronchopulmonary infection with *Pseudomonas aeruginosa. J. Clin. Invest.* **100**, 2810-2815 (1997).

18. U. Sajjan, G. Thanassoulis, V. Cherapanov, A. Lu, C. Sjolin, B. Steer, Y.J. Wu, O.D. Rotstein, G. Kent, C. McKerlie, J. Forstner, and P. Downey. Enhanced susceptibility to pulmonary infection with *Burkholderia cepacia* in *Cftr*$^{-/-}$ mice. *Infect. Immun.* **69**, 5138-5150 (2001).

19. D. Oceandy, B.J. McMorran, S.N. Smith, R. Schreiber, K. Kunzelmann, E.W. Alton, D.A. Hume, and B.J. Wainwright. Gene complementation of airway epithelium in the cystic fibrosis mouse is necessary and sufficient to correct the pathogen clearance and inflammatory abnormalities. *Hum. Mol. Genet.* **11**, 1059-1067 (2002).

20. G. Lamblin, S. Degroote, J.-M. Perini, P. Delmotte, A. Scharfman, M. Davril, J.-M. Lo-Guidice, N. Houdret, V. Dumur, A. Klein, and P. Roussel. Human airway mucin glycosylation: a combinatory of carbohydrate determinants which vary in Cystic Fibrosis. *Glycoconj. J.* **18**, 661-684 (2001).

21. V. Debailleul, A. Laine, G. Huet, P. Mathon, M.C. d'Hooghe, J.-P. Aubert, and N. Porchet. Human mucin genes *MUC2, MUC3, MUC4, MUC5AC, MUC5B,* and *MUC6*

express stable and extremely large mRNAs and exhibit a variable length polymorphism - an improved method to analyze large mRNAs. *J. Biol. Chem.* **273**, 881-890 (1998).

22. N. Moniaux, F. Escande, N. Porchet, J.-P. Aubert, and S.K. Batra. Structural organization and classification of the mucin genes. *Front. Biosci.* **6**, d1192-1206 (2001).

23. S.J. Williams, D.H. Wreschner, M. Tran, H.J. Eyre, G.R. Sutherland, and M.A. McGuckin. Muc13, a novel human cell surface mucin expressed by epithelial and hemopoietic cells. *J. Biol. Chem.* **276**, 18327-18336 (2001).

24. Y. Chen, Y.H. Zhao, T.B. Kalaslavadi, E. Hamati, K. Nehrke, A.D. Le, D.K. Ann, and R. Wu. Genome-wide search and identification of a novel gel-forming mucin MUC19/Muc19 in glandular tissues. *Am. J. Respir. Cell Mol. Biol.* **30**, 155-165 (2004).

25. J.F. Engelhardt, J.R. Yankaskas, S.A. Ernst, Y. Yang, C.R. Marino, R.C. Boucher, J.A. Cohn, and J.M. Wilson. Submucosal glands are the predominant site of CFTR expression in the human bronchus. *Nat. Genet.* **3**, 240-248 (1992).

26. J.F. Engelhardt, M. Zepeda, J.A. Cohn, J.R. Yankaskas, and J.M. Wilson. Expression of the cystic fibrosis gene in adult human lung. *J. Clin. Invest.* **93**, 737-749 (1994).

27. J. Jacquot, E. Puchelle, J. Hinnrasky, C. Fuchey, C. Bettinger, C. Spilmont, N. Bonnet, A. Dieterle, D. Dreyer, A. Pavirani *et al.* Localization of the cystic fibrosis transmembrane conductance regulator in airway secretory glands. *Eur. Respir. J.* **6**, 169-176 (1993).

28. Y. Chen, Y. H. Zhao, Y.-P. Di, and R. Wu. Characterization of human Mucin 5B gene expression in airway epithelium and its genomic clone of the amino-terminal and 5'-flanking region. *Am. J. Respir. Cell Mol. Biol.* **2**, 5542-5553 (2001).

29. M. Zuhdi Alimam, F.M. Piazza, D.M. Selby, N. Letwin, L. Huang, and M.C. Rose. Muc-5/5ac mucin messenger RNA and protein expression is a marker of goblet cell metaplasia in murine airways, *Am. J. Respir. Cell Mol. Biol.* **22**, 253-260 (2000).

30. P. Delmotte, S. Degroote, M.D. Merten, I. Van Seuningen, A. Bernigaud, C. Figarella, P. Roussel, and J.-M. Perini. Influence of TNFalpha on the sialylation of mucins produced by a transformed cell line MM-39 derived from human tracheal gland cells. *Glycoconj. J.* **18**, 487-497 (2001).

31. Y. Chen, P. Thai, Y.H. Zhao, Y.S. Ho, M.M. DeSouza, and R. Wu. Stimulation of airway mucin gene expression by interleukin (IL)-17 through IL-6 paracrine/autocrine loop. *J. Biol. Chem.* **278**, 17036-17043 (2003).

32. M.T. Borchers, M.P. Carty, and G.D. Leikauf. Regulation of human airway mucins by acrolein and inflammatory mediators. *Am. J. Physiol.* **276**, L549-555 (1999).

33. S.J. Levine, P. Larivee, C. Logun, C.W. Angus, F.P. Ognibene, and J.H. Shelhamer. Tumor necrosis factor-α induces mucin hypersecretion and *MUC-2* gene expression by human airway epithelial cells. *Am. J. Respir. Cell. Mol. Biol.* **12**, 196-204 (1995).

34. J. Iwashita, Y. Sato, H. Sugaya, N. Takahashi, H. Sasaki, and T. Abe. mRNA of MUC2 is stimulated by IL-4, IL-13 or TNF-alpha through a mitogen-activated protein kinase pathway in human colon cancer cells. *Immunol. Cell Biol.* **81**, 275-282 (2003).

35. J.S. Koo, Y.D. Kim, A.M. Jetten, P. Belloni, and P. Nettesheim. Overexpression of mucin genes induced by interleukin-1 beta, tumor necrosis factor-alpha, lipopolysaccharide, and neutrophil elastase is inhibited by a retinoic acid receptor alpha antagonist. *Exp. Lung Res.* **28**, 315-332 (2002).

36. U.A. Temann, B. Prasad, M.W. Gallup, C. Basbaum, S.B. Ho, R. A. Flavell, and J.A. Rankin. A novel role for murine IL-4 in vivo: induction of MUC5AC gene expression and mucin hypersecretion. *Am. J. Respir. Cell Mol. Biol.* **16**, 471-478 (1997).

37. K. Dabbagh, K. Takeyama, H.M. Lee, I.F. Ueki, J.A. Lausier, and J.A. Nadel. IL-4 induces mucin gene expression and goblet cell metaplasia *in vitro* and *in vivo*. *J. Immunol.* **162**, 6233-6237 (1999).

38. M. Longphre, D. Li, M. Gallup, L. Drori, C.L. Ordonez, T. Redman, S. Wenzel, D.E. Bice, J.V. Fahy, and C. Basbaum. Allergen-induced IL-9 directly stimulates mucin transcription in epithelial cells. *J. Clin. Invest.* **104**, 1375-1382 (1999).

39. J. Louahed, M. Toda, J. Jen, Q. Hamid, J.C. Renauld, R.C. Levitt, and N.C. Nicolaides. Interleukin-9 upregulates mucus expression in the airways. *Am. J. Respir. Cell. Mol. Biol.* **22**, 649-56 (2000).

40. J.R.Reader, D.M. Hyde, E.S. Schelegle, M.C. Aldrich, A.M. Stoddard, M.P. McLane, R.C. Levitt, and J.S. Tepper. Interleukin-9 induces mucous cell metaplasia independent of inflammation *Am. J. Respir. Cell Mol. Biol.* **28**, 664-672 (2003).

41. M. Perrais, P. Pigny, M.-C. Copin, J.-P. Aubert, and I. Van Seuningen. Induction of MUC2 and MUC5AC mucins by factors of the epidermal growth factor (EGF) family is mediated by EGF receptor/Ras/Raf/extracellular signal-regulated kinase cascade and Sp1. *J. Biol. Chem.* **277**, 32258-32267 (2002).

42. N. McNamara and C. Basbaum. Signaling networks controlling mucin production in response to Gram-positive and Gram-negative bacteria. *Glycoconj. J.* **18**, 715-722 (2001).

43. K. Takeyama, B. Jung, J.J. Shim, P.R. Burgel, T. Dao-Piçk, I.F. Ueki, U. Protin, P. Kroschel, and J.A. Nadel. Activation of epidermal growth factor receptors is responsible for mucin synthesis induced by cigarette smoke. *Am. J. Physiol. Lung Cell Mol. Physiol.* **280**, L165-172 (2001).

44. M.A. McPherson, M.M. Pereira, D. Russell, C.M. McNeilly, R.M. Morris, F.L. Stratford, and R.L. Dormer. The CFTR-mediated protein secretion defect: pharmacological correction. *Pflugers Arch.* **443** Suppl 1, S121-126 (2001).

45. J. Perez-Vilar, S.H. Randell, and R. Boucher. The cys subdomains of human gel-forming mucins are C-mannosylated domains involved in weak protein-protein interactions. *Ped. Pulmonol.* **24** suppl, 190 (2002).

46. W. Morelle, M. Sutton-Smith, H.R. Morris, M. Davril, P. Roussel, and A. Dell. FAB-MS characterization of sialyl Lewis^x determinants on polylactosamine chains of human airway mucins secreted by patients suffering from cystic fibrosis or chronic bronchitis. *Glycoconj. J.* **18**, 699-708 (2001).

47. K.A. Thomsson, I. Carlstedt, N.G. Karlsson, H. Karlsson, and G.C. Hansson. Different O-glycosylation of respiratory mucin glycopeptides from a patient with cystic fibrosis. *Glycoconj. J.* **15**, 823-833 (1998).

48. T.W. De Graaf, M.E. Van der Stelt, M.G. Anbergen, and W. van Dijk. Inflammation-induced expression of sialyl-Lewis X-containing glycan structures on α_1-acid glycoprotein (orosomucoid) in human sera. *J. Exp. Med.* **177**, 657-666 (1993).

49. M. Davril, S. Degroote, P. Humbert, C. Galabert, V. Dumur, J.-J. Lafitte, G. Lamblin, and P. Roussel. The sialylation of bronchial mucins secreted by patients suffering from cystic fibrosis or from chronic bronchitis is related to the severity of airway infection. *Glycobiology* **9**, 311-321 (1999).

50. G. Lamblin, J.-J. Lafitte, M. Lhermitte, P. Degand, and P. Roussel. Mucins from cystic fibrosis sputum. *Mod. Probl. Paediat.* **19**, 153-164 (1977).

51. K.V. Chace, M. Flux, and G.P. Sachdev. Comparison of physicochemical properties of purified mucus glycoproteins isolated from respiratory secretions of cystic fibrosis and asthmatic patients. *Biochemistry* **24**, 7334-7341 (1985).

52. R.C. Frates Jr, T.T. Kaizu, and J.A. Last. Mucus glycoproteins secreted by respiratory epithelial tissue from cystic fibrosis patients. *Pediatr. Res.* **17**, 30-34 (1983).

53. Y. Zhang, B. Doranz, J.R. Yankaskas, and J.F. Engelhardt. Genotypic analysis of respiratory mucous sulfation defects in cystic fibrosis. *J. Clin. Invest.* **96**, 2997-3004 (1995).

54. C. Carnoy, R. Ramphal, A. Scharfman, N. Houdret, J.-M. Lo-Guidice, A. Klein, C. Galabert, G. Lamblin, and P. Roussel. Altered carbohydrate composition of salivary mucins from patients with cystic fibrosis and the adhesion of *Pseudomonas aeruginosa*. *Am. J. Respir. Cell. Mol. Biol.* **9**, 323-334 (1993).

55. D.K. Shori, T. Genter, J. Hansen, C. Koch, H. Wyatt, H.H. Kariyawasam, R.A. Knight, M.E. Hodson, A. Kalogeridis, and I. Tsanakas. Altered sialyl- and fucosyl-linkage on mucins in cystic fibrosis patients promotes formation of the sialyl-Lewis X determinant on salivary MUC-5B and MUC-7. *Pflugers Arch.* **443** Suppl, S55-61 (2001).

56. J.-M. Lo-Guidice, J.-M. Wieruszewski, J. Lemoine, A. Verbert, P. Roussel, and G. Lamblin. Sialylation and sulfation of the carbohydrate chains in respiratory mucins from a patient with cystic fibrosis. *J. Biol. Chem.* **269**, 18794-18813 (1994).

57. J.-M. Lo-Guidice, M. Herz, G. Lamblin, Y. Plancke, P. Roussel, and M. Lhermitte. Structures of sulfated oligosaccharides isolated from the respiratory mucins of a non-secretor (O, Le^{a+b-}) patient suffering from chronic bronchitis. *Glycoconj. J.* **14**, 113-125 (1997).

58. S. Degroote, E. Maes, P. Humbert, P. Delmotte, G. Lamblin, and P. Roussel. Sulfated oligosaccharides isolated from the respiratory mucins of a secretor patient suffering from chronic bronchitis. *Biochimie* **85**, 369-379 (2003).

59. N.W. Lukacs, R.M. Strieter, S.W. Chensue, M. Widmer, and S.L. Kunkel. TNF-alpha mediates recruitment of neutrophils and eosinophils during airway inflammation. *J. Immunol.* **154**, 5411-5417 (1995).

60. E. Osika, J.-M. Cavaillon, K. Chadelat, M. Boule, C. Fitting, G. Tournier, and A. Clement. Distinct sputum cytokine profiles in cystic fibrosis and other chronic inflammatory airway disease. *Eur. Respir. J.* **14**, 339-346 (1999).

61. F. Karpati, F.L. Hjelte, and B. Wretlind. TNF-alpha and IL-8 in consecutive sputum samples from cystic fibrosis patients during antibiotic treatment. *Scand. J. Infect. Dis.* **32**, 75-79 (2000).

62. P. Delmotte, S. Degroote, J.-J. Lafitte, G. Lamblin, J.-M. Perini, and P. Roussel. Tumor necrosis factor alpha increases the expression of glycosyltransferases and sulfotransferases responsible for the biosynthesis of sialylated and/or sulfated Lewis x epitopes in the human bronchial mucosa. *J. Biol. Chem.* **277**, 424-431 (2002).

63. J.N. Couceiro, J.C. Paulson, and L.G. Baum. Influenza virus strains selectively recognize sialyloligosaccharides on human respiratory epithelium: the role of the host cell in selection of hemagglutinin receptor specificity. *Virus Res.* **29**, 155-165 (1993).

64. A. Dosanjh, W. Lencer, D. Brown, D.A. Ausiello, and J.L. Stow. Heterologous expression of ΔF508 CFTR results in decreased sialylation of membrane glycoconjugates. *Am. J. Physiol.* **266**, C360-C366 (1994).

65. J. Barasch, B. Kiss, A. Prince, L. Saiman, D. Gruenert, and Q. Al-Awqati. Defective acidification of intracellular organelles in cystic fibrosis. *Nature* **352**, 70-73 (1991).

66. M.C. Glick, V.A. Kothari, A. Liu, L.I. Stoykova, and T.F. Scanlin. Activity of fucosyltransferases and altered glycosylation in cystic fibrosis airway epithelial cells. *Biochimie* **83**, 743-747 (2001).

67. P.W. Cheng, T.F. Boat, K. Cranfill, J.R. Yankaskas, and R.C. Boucher. Increased sulfation of glycoconjugates by cultured nasal epithelial cells from patients with cystic fibrosis. *J. Clin. Invest.* **84**, 68-72 (1989).

68. N.K. Mohapatra, P.W. Cheng, J.C. Parker, A.M. Paradiso, J.R. Yankaskas, R.C. Boucher, and T.F. Boat. Alteration of sulfation of glycoconjugates, but not sulfate transport and intracellular inorganic sulfate content in cystic fibrosis airway epithelial cells. *Pediatr. Res.* **38**, 42-48 (1995).

69. J. Barasch and Q. Al-Awqati. Defective acidification of the biosynthetic pathway in cystic fibrosis. *J. Cell Sci. Suppl.* **17**, 229-233 (1993).

70. O. Seksek, J. Biwersi, and A.S. Verkman. Evidence against defective *trans*-Golgi acidification in cystic fibrosis. *J. Biol. Chem.* **271**, 15542-15548 (1996).

71. J.F. Poschet, J.C. Boucher, L. Tatterson, J. Skidmore, R.W. Van Dyke, and V. Deretic. Molecular basis for defective glycosylation and *Pseudomonas* pathogenesis in cystic fibrosis lung. *Proc. Natl. Acad. Sci. U.S.A.* **98**, 13972-13977 (2001).

72. E.A. Pasyk and J.K. Foskett. Cystic fibrosis transmembrane conductance regulator-associated ATP and adenosine 3'-phosphate 5'-phosphosulfate channels in endoplasmic reticulum and plasma membranes. *J. Biol. Chem.* **272**, 7746-7751 (1997).

73. S. De Bentzmann, P. Roger, F. Dupuit, O. Bajolet-Laudinat, C. Fuchey, M.C. Plotkowski, and E. Puchelle. Asialo GM1 is a receptor for *Pseudomonas aeruginosa* adherence to regenerating respiratory epithelial cells. *Infect. Immun.* **64**, 1582-1588 (1996).

74. L. Saiman and A. Prince. *Pseudomonas aeruginosa* pili binds asialo-GM1 which is increased at the surface of cystic fibrosis epithelial cells. *J. Clin. Invest.* **92**, 187?-1880 (1993).

75. D.L. Simel, J.P. Mastin, P.C. Pratt, C.L. Wisseman, J.D. Shelburne, A. Spock, and P. Ingram. Scanning electron microscopic study of the airways in normal children and in patients with cystic fibrosis and other lung diseases. *Pediatr. Pathol.* **2**, 47-64 (1984).

76. P.K. Jeffrey and A.P.R. Brain. Surface morphology of human airway mucosa: Normal, carcinoma or cystic fibrosis. *Scanning Microsc.* **2**, 345-351 (1988).

77. R. Ramphal, P.M. Small, J.W. Shands Jr, W. Fischlschweiger, and P.A. Small. Adherence of *Pseudomonas aeruginosa* to tracheal cells injured by influenza infection or by endotracheal intubation. *Infect. Immun.* **27**, 614-619 (1980).

78. H.C. Krivan, V. Ginsburg, and D.D. Roberts, *Pseudomonas aeruginosa* and *Pseudomonas cepacia* isolated from cystic fibrosis patients bind specifically to gangliotetraosylceramide (asialo GM1) and gangliotriaosylceramide (asialo GM2). *Arch. Biochem. Biophys.* **260**, 493-496 (1988).

79. H.B. Sheth, K.K. Lee, W.Y. Wong, G. Srivastava, O. Hindsgaul, R.S. Hodges, W. Paranchych, and R.T. Irvin. The pili of *Pseudomonas aeruginosa* strains PAK and PAO bind specifically to the carbohydrate sequence beta GalNAc(1-4)betaGal found in glycosphingolipids asialo-GM1 and asialo-GM2. *Mol. Microbiol.* **11**, 715-23 (1994).

80. R. Ramphal and S.K. Arora. Recognition of mucin components by *Pseudomonas aeruginosa*. *Glycoconj. J.* **18**, 709-713 (2001).

81. N. Devaraj, M. Sheykhnazari, W.S. Warren, and V.P. Bhavanandan. Differential binding of *Pseudomonas aeruginosa* to normal and cystic fibrosis tracheobronchial mucins. *Glycobiology* **4**, 307-316 (1994).

82. C. Carnoy, A. Scharfman, E. Van Brussel, G. Lamblin, R. Ramphal, and P. Roussel. *Pseudomonas aeruginosa* outer membrane adhesins for human respiratory mucus glycoproteins. *Infect. Immun.* **62**, 1896-1900 (1994).

83. R. Ramphal, L. Koo, K.S. Ishimoto, P.A. Totten, J.C. Lara, and S. Lory. Adhesion of *Pseudomonas aeruginosa* pilin-deficient mutants to mucin. *Infect. Immun.* **59**, 1307-1311 (1991).

84. R. Ramphal, N. Houdret, L. Koo, G. Lamblin, and P. Roussel. Differences in adhesion of *Pseudomonas aeruginosa* to mucin glycopeptides from sputa of patients with cystic fibrosis and chronic bronchitis. *Infect. Immun.* **57**, 3066-3071 (1989).

85. S.K. Arora, B.W. Ritchings, E.C. Almira, S. Lory, and R. Ramphal. The *Pseudomonas aeruginosa* flagellar cap protein, FliD, is responsible for mucin adhesion. *Infect. Immun.* **66**, 1000-1007 (1998).

86. A. Scharfman, S.K. Arora, P. Delmotte, E. Van Brussel, J. Mazurier, R. Ramphal, and P. Roussel. Recognition of Lewis x derivatives present on mucins by flagellar components of *Pseudomonas aeruginosa*. *Infect .Immun.* **69**, 5243-8 (2001).

87. R. Ramphal, C. Carnoy, S. Fievre, J.-C. Michalski, N. Houdret, G. Lamblin, G. Strecker, and P. Roussel. *Pseudomonas aeruginosa* recognizes carbohydrate chains containing type 1 (Galβ1-3GlcNAc) or type 2 (Galβ1-4GlcNAc) disaccharide units. *Infect. Immun.* **59**, 700-704 (1991).

88. I.J. Rosenstein, C.T. Yuen, M.S. Stoll, and T. Feizi. Differences in the binding specificities of *Pseudomonas aeruginosa* M35 and *Escherichia coli* C600 for lipid-linked oligosaccharides with lactose-related core regions. *Infect. Immun.* **60**, 5078-5084 (1992).

89. A. Scharfman, S. Degroote, J. Beau, G. Lamblin, P. Roussel, and J. Mazurier. *Pseudomonas aeruginosa* binds to neoglycoconjugates bearing mucin carbohydrate determinants and predominantly to sialyl-Lewis x conjugates. *Glycobiology* **9**, 757-764 (1999).

90. A. Scharfman, P. Delmotte, J. Beau, G. Lamblin, P. Roussel, and J. Mazurier. Sialyl-Le(x) and sulfo-sialyl-Le(x) determinants are receptors for *P. aeruginosa*. *Glycoconj. J.* **10**, 735-740 (2000).

91. H. Rahmoune, G. Lamblin, J.-J. Lafitte, C. Galabert, M. Filliat, and P. Roussel. Chondroitin sulfate in sputum from patients with cystic fibrosis and chronic bronchitis. *Am. J. Respir. Cell Mol. Biol.* **5**, 315-320 (1991).

92. I.A. Khatri, R. Bhaskar, J.T. Lamont, S.U. Sajjan, C.K. Y. Ho, and J. Forstner. Effect of chondroitinase ABC on purulent sputum from cystic fibrosis and other patients. *Pediatr. Res.* **53**, 619-627 (2003).

93. M.C. Brahimi-Horn, E. Deudon, A. Paul, M. Mergey, C. Mailleau, C. Basbaum, A. Dohrman, and J. Capeau. Identification of decorin proteoglycan in bovine tracheal serous cells in culture and localization of decorin mRNA in situ. *Eur. J. Cell Biol.* **64**, 271-280 (1994).

94. B. Rasche, K. Hochstrasser, and W.T. Ulmer. Inter-alpha-trypsin inhibitor in serum and bronchial mucus inhibitor in sputum in chronic airway obstruction. *Respiration* **36**, 39-47 (1978).

95. T.S. Blackwell, A.A. Stecenko, and J.W. Christman. Dysregulated NF-κB activation in cystic fibrosis: evidence for a primary inflammatory disorder. *Am. J. Physiol. Lung Cell. Mol. Physiol.* **281**, L69-70 (2001).

Chapter 12

BIOSYNTHESIS AND SECRETION OF MUCINS, ESPECIALLY THE MUC2 MUCIN, IN RELATION TO CYSTIC FIBROSIS

Gunnar C. Hansson, Malin E.V. Johansson, and Martin E. Lidell
Department of Medical Biochemistry, Göteborg University, Medicinaregatan 9A 413 90 Gothenburg, Sweden. Tel: +46-31-7733488, Fax: +46-31-416108 ; E-mail: gunnar.hansson@medkem.gu.se

1.   INTRODUCTION

The mucosal surfaces of the body are not protected by several layers of dead cells as is the case for the skin. Instead, the mucosal surfaces are protected by mucus. The major function of this mucus layer is to protect the epithelial cells, to trap and to transport foreign material as microorganisms away. The properties of this mucus has to be delicately balanced, something that is especially difficult in the intestine where the mucus has to allow digested nutrients to pass and at the same time withstand the digestive enzymes.

Cystic fibrosis (CF) is characterized by a dysfunctional CFTR channel.[1] In addition to the salt loosing character of CF that is easy to correlate with the absence of functional CFTR chloride channels, the sticky and viscous mucus is the most easily recognized property of this disease. However, despite that 15 years has passed since the discovery of CFTR, it has been difficult to find a convincing explanation for this relation. Studies made possible by the human bronchial epithelial (HBE) cultures grown at an air-liquid interface has changed this and solved at least part of the puzzle. When the liquid between the apical surface of the ciliated cells and the mucus layer were measured *in vivo* using confocal microscopy, it turned out that also after the addition of extra liquid, the height of this so called apical surface liquid (ASL) was considerably lower on CF as compared to normal cells.[2] This causes the mucus to fall down onto the cilia of the epithelial cells and the mucus is trapped and cannot move. This is illustrated by the very limited movement of the mucus on the CF HBE cultures as compared to cultures from normal donors. That the ASL do not distance the mucus gel to far from the cilia is also important as it will result in poor clearance. Thus it is very important to have an ASL of the right height. It is suggested that CFTR is an important regulator of the ASL height and that a non-functional CFTR causes mucus trapping.

2.   MUCINS

Mucins are large and highly glycosylated proteins found at mucosal surfaces. The mucins are characterized by the mucin or PTS domains due to the abundant amino acids Pro, Thr and Ser. These are often arranged in tandem repeats and frequently show polymorphism between individuals both in number of repeats and sequence. The hydroxy amino acids serve as attachment sites for the high-density O-glycosylation, giving the mucin domains an extended 'bottle brush' like structure. These mucin domains dominate the mucin molecules, although these domains can be found also in other proteins predominantly at the cell surface. Because of the large size of the mucin domains, the carbohydrates make up most of the mass, often exceeding 80%.

There are two major groups of mucins, the transmembrane and polymeric mucins. In addition, there is at least one secreted monomeric mucin called MUC7. In higher animals, the transmembrane mucins are predominant in number. These mucins have a large extracellular, mucin domain followed by a stalk region, a transmembrane part and a cytoplasmic tail. The human transmembrane mucins are MUC1, MUC3A, MUC3B, MUC4, MUC12, MUC13, MUC16, and MUC17. The other major group of mucins is the polymeric gel-forming ones. There are five known mucins of this group in the human genome, MUC2, MUC5AC, MUC5B, MUC6 and MUC19, all showing large sequence similarities in their N- and C-termini. The MUC2 mucin will be discussed here as an example of such a molecule.

3.   THE MUC2 MUCIN

The MUC2 mucin is the predominant mucin in the small and large intestine. This mucin has two mucin domains, one small (382 amino acids) and one large (2310 amino acids), that together with a small Cys-rich domain (called CysD domain) make up the central half of the protein as outlined in Figure 1. Both the N- and C-termini are rich in the amino acid Cys and contain four von Willebrand D domains (three in the N- and one in the C-terminus). The most C-terminal part is made up of a CK domain, involved in dimerization. These termini are highly homologous to the other gel-forming mucins and the von Willebrand factor involved in blood coagulation. All these molecules are assembled into larger polymers using these N- and C-termini. The MUC2 mucin is made up of a total of 5179 amino acids and is thus, already before glycosylation, a large protein. The assembly of MUC2 has been studied by us and the current understanding is discussed below.

3.1   Assembly of the MUC2 mucin

The assembly of MUC2 will be followed through the secretory pathway and reflect our knowledge obtained both form native MUC2 (in LS 174T cells) and the expression of truncated recombinant constructs in CHO and LS 174T cells.[3-8] The primary translational product of full length MUC2 or recombinant C-terminus is quickly **dimerized in the endoplasmic reticulum (ER)**. The definite proof that the C-terminus forms dimers have recently been obtained by molecular electron microscopy showing the recombinant MUC2 C-terminal dimers attached **end to end.**[7]

After the ER, the dimers pass into the Golgi apparatus, where O-glycosylation takes place and the mass increases to about 5 MDa. Some non-dimerized monomers also pass into the Golgi apparatus. In pulse-chase studies, the glycosylated dimers then quickly become insoluble, but not the monomers, and are found in the pellet after centrifugation. This insoluble MUC2 can be recovered by disulfide-bond reduction of this pellet.[5] The disappearance of the MUC2 into an insoluble product made further progress in elucidating the assembly of MUC2 using the native, full-length MUC2 impossible. When the insoluble MUC2 was analyzed after disulfide-bond reduction, not only the expected monomers were observed, but also non-reducible dimers were found, suggesting that these are held together by covalent, non-disulfide bonds. This is similar to an early observation by Carlstedt et al., where the MUC2 recovered from the intestine was found to be insoluble in guanidinium chloride and that this also contained non-reducible oligomers.[9, 10] The nature of this suggested non-reducible linkage is still not known.

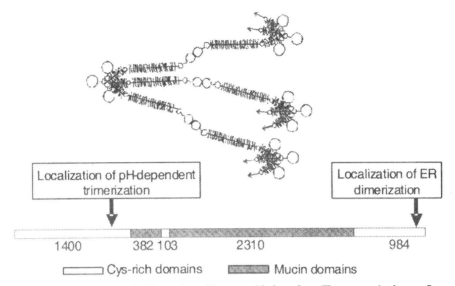

Figure 1. Model of the MUC2 mucin and its assembled product. The arrows in the top figure indicate where the assembled protein is further extended.

To overcome the problems caused by the MUC2 protein becoming insoluble, we turned to the expression of recombinant truncated forms of MUC2. The N-terminal construct was made with the green fluorescent protein (EGFP) and a myc-Tag inserted instead of the central mucin domains. When the N-terminus was expressed in CHO cells, a disulfide-bond stabilized oligomer larger than a dimer was secreted. We could recently reveal that these were without doubt **trimers**. This was shown by several lines of evidence, where the electron microscopy pictures was the final convincing evidence[6].This was not expected as mucins have been predicted to be linear polymers, as the homologous polymeric protein, the von Willebrand factor. This trimerization probably takes place in the secretory vesicles and is blocked by neutralization of the low pH in this part of the secretory pathway.

The studies performed suggest a model for the MUC2 structure as is outlined in Figure 1, where the MUC2 mucin is forming large net-like polymeric structures.

3.2   Non-enzymatic cleavage

Recently we found a non-enzymatic, autocatalytic cleavage in the MUC2 C-terminus. This was first observed during the preparation of the recombinant C-terminus as expressed in CHO cells. When the dimers were separated at low pH, the C-terminus was observed cleaved into two smaller fragments. This cleavage turned out to be identical to the beginning of a MUC2 C-terminal fragment previously observed by Forstner *et al.* and called the 'link peptide'.[11] The MUC2 **C-terminus** is cleaved at the GD/PH sequence by a non-enzymatic autocatalytic mechanism triggered by low pH.[12] The elucidation of this cleavage is illustrated in Fig. 2. This cleavage was observed both *in vitro* and *in vivo*, where it could be inhibited by neutralizing the secretory pathway.[12] We have also shown that an internal anhydride was generated in the newly formed C-terminal Asp. This type of anhydride is very reactive and is able to react with primary amines or hydroxy groups. In fact, we have been able to show that a biotinylated primary amine reacts and covalently attaches to this new C-terminus. The MUC5AC mucin is the only additional gel-forming mucin that contains the GDPH sequence and we suggest that this mucin is also cleaved in an analogous way generating a reactive new C-terminus. The MUC5AC mucin is together with MUC5B the main mucins of the lung.

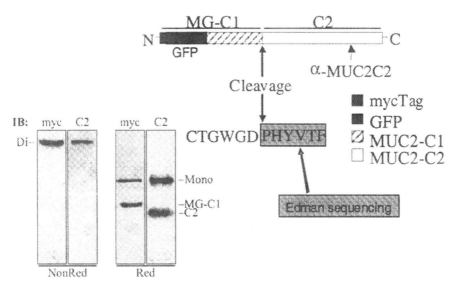

Figure 2. Experimental evidence for the cleavage of the C-terminus of MUC2 as shown by the expression of a recombinant MUC2 fusion protein. The localization of the cleavage was determined by Edman sequencing and the fragments obtained characterized by polyacrylamide gel electrophoresis and western blot with antibodies as indicated.

4.   GEL-FORMING MUCINS AND CYSTIC FIBROSIS

In addition to the low ASL thickness, if there is any biochemical reasons to the adherent and viscous mucus found at CF these should most likely be sought among the mucins. The gel-forming ones are discussed here, but there are some indications for the involvement of the transmembrane mucins. We have shown that MUC1 is upregulated in the intestine of CF mice due to the expression of alternative splice variants of which one has not been observed before.[13, 14] In contrast to this, little progress has been made in revealing a potential role of the gel-forming mucins in the CF pathology during the years and progress is in high demand. Here we propose two mechanisms that could be involved.

4.1   Is MUC2 expressed in the CF lungs part of the CF phenotype?

The normal lung produces two gel-forming mucins, the MUC5AC in the goblet cells and the MUC5B in the glands. However, under pathological conditions the MUC2 mucin has also been detected in the lungs, both at the transcriptional and protein levels.[15-17] The transcriptional activation of MUC2 by the common CF pathogen *Pseudomonas aeruginosa* has been shown to be mediated via the NFκB pathway.

The properties of the MUC2 mucin are adapted to resist the harsh milieu in the intestine. This is reflected in its insolubility as discussed above, a property not found to any appreciable degree in the MUC5AC and MUC5B mucins from the lungs,[16] but well noted for MUC5B in saliva.[18] The lung mucins are adapted for mucus clearance as mediated by the cilia transportation, but the properties of MUC2 might cause transportation difficulties and cause retention in the lung. This scenario could be envisaged by the observations by Davies *et al.* who detected only small amounts (<4% of the mucins) of MUC2 in the sputa of CF patients, whereas the transcriptional studies suggested that MUC2 mucin should be relatively abundant. It can be speculated that the induction of MUC2 is part of a second defense mechanism, causing no detrimental effects if the lungs recover as for non-CF individuals. However, this could be detrimental for CF patients and part of the problems with the chronic infection typical for the CF lung phenotype. To further address this question, it should be important to compare the levels of MUC2 protein in the lungs and sputa and by this elucidate if MUC2 is only a very minor component as suggested from studies of CF sputa [16] or if there is a selective retention of MUC2 in the lungs.

4.2   Anchoring of mucins to epithelial cells?

The autocatalytic cleavage of MUC2, and possibly MUC5AC, as discussed above can take place in the later, more acidic parts of the secretory pathway of cells with a regulated secretory pathway. This is exemplified by the cell line LS 174T [12] that contains large goblet cell-like granulae. It is a relatively safe to assume that MUC2 is cleaved in these storage granulae of goblet cells of the intestine as a substantial portion of the MUC2 isolated from the intestine has been shown to be cleaved.[10] However, it is currently not known if the generated anhydride has reacted with a specific target or not. Our studies have shown that the cleavage is relatively slow and can approach 50% after 24 hours. This suggests that MUC2, also after normal storage in goblet cells, should not be cleaved to 100%. Thus uncleaved MUC2 should be found in the extracellular mucus and have the possibility to undergo further cleavage if the appropriate acidic conditions are found. This is probably especially relevant for CF as the ASL has recently been shown to be more acidic than normal.[19] The CF cells have an impaired response to acidification of the ASL and show a pH about 0.5 units lower than normal. The ASL in CF can have a pH can approaching pH 6, an acidic milieu sufficient for triggering the cleavage of at least MUC2. As MUC5AC contains the same cleavable sequence, it is likely that also this normal respiratory mucin can be cleaved. The CF ASL is also characterized by being considerably thinner, not allowing the mucus gel to float on the cilia. The mucus will thus be in close contact with the cilia and epithelial cells where the generation of Asp anhydrides by cleavages in MUC5AC and MUC2 could be envisioned to react and attach the mucus to any free amine or hydroxyl group. These groups could of course be found on other gel-forming mucins or soluble proteins in the gel, but also in the epithelially anchored molecules. The mucin gel could thus be covalently attached to the epithelial cells. This scenario is outlined in Fig. 3.

A similar scenario can also be suggested for the intestine, although no experimental results support a thinner liquid layer between the epithelial cells and the mucus layer. That this is really the case is suggested by some CF patients having problem with intestinal obstruction and an adherent intestinal content. This is similar to the meconium ileus, a common problem of newborn CF children. A lower pH in the intestine of CF patients has been observed, but has been believed to be due to the lack of HCO_3^- secretion from the pancreas. A hypothesis similar to the one for the respiratory tract (Fig. 3) where the mucus gel is more firmly attached to the epithelial cells can thus be raised also in the case for the intestine.

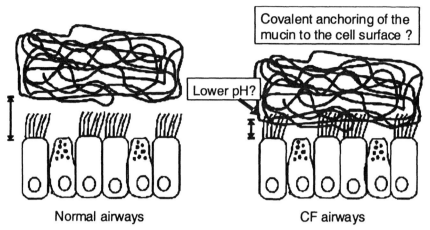

Figure 3. Schematic picture showing a potential scenario for the attachment of mucus the ciliated cells of CF patients.

5.   CONCLUDING REMARKS

The typical CF symptoms with viscous and trapped mucus are still lacking a full explanation. Here we suggest that the CF mucus become sticky and adherent to the epithelial cells by a covalent attachment of MUC2 and MUC5AC. We also suggest that the expression of MUC2 in the lungs could contribute to the CF phenotype. However, there are several unanswered questions before these suggestions can be proved. Among the most urgent ones are to show to what molecules the generated anhydride can attach or if the anhydride only has been hydrolyzed. Once this and other questions have been answered, one can start to address potential therapeutic approaches using recent advances in mucin knowledge.

ACKNOWLEDGMENTS

The work discussed here was supported by the Swedish Research Council and the Swedish Cystic Fibrosis Foundation.

REFERENCES

1. J. R. Riordan, J. M. Rommens, B. S. Kerem, N. Alon, R. Rozmahel, Z. Grzelczak, J. Zielenski, S. Lok, N. Plavsic, J. L. Chou, M. L. Drumm, M. C. Iannuzzi, F. S. Collins, and

L. C. Tsui, Identification of the cystic fibrosis gene: Cloning and characterization of complementary DNA, *Science* **245**, 1066-1072 (1989).

2. H. Matsui, B. R. Grubb, R. Tarran, S. H. Randell, J. T. Gatzy, C. W. Davis, and R. C. Boucher, Evidence for periciliary liqulid layer depletion, not abnormal ion composition, in the pathogenesis of cystic fibrosis airways disease, *Cell* **95**, 1005-1015 (1998).

3. N. Asker, D. Baeckstrom, M. A. B. Axelsson, I. Carlstedt, and G. C. Hansson, The human MUC2 mucin apoprotein appears to dimerize before O-glycosylation and shares epitopes with the 'insoluble' mucin of rat small intestine, *Biochem. J.* **308**, 873-880 (1995).

4. N. Asker, M. A. B. Axelsson, S. O. Olofsson, and G. C. Hansson, Dimerization of the human MUC2 mucin in the endoplasmic reticulum is followed by a N-glycosylation-dependent transfer of the mono- and dimers to the Golgi apparatus, *J. Biol. Chem.* **273**, 18857-18863 (1998).

5. M. A. B. Axelsson, N. Asker, and G. C. Hansson, O-glycosylated MUC2 monomer and dimer from LS 174T cells are water-soluble, whereas larger MUC2 species formed early during biosynthesis are insoluble and contain nonreducible intermolecular bonds, *J. Biol. Chem.* **273**, 18864-18870 (1998).

6. K. Godl, M. E. V. Johansson, H. Karlsson, M. Morgelin, M. E. Lidell, F. J. Olson, J. R. Gum, Y. S. Kim, and G. C. Hansson, The N-termini of the MUC2 mucin form trimers that are held together within a trypsin-resistant core fragment, *J. Biol. Chem.* **277**, 47248-47256 (2002).

7. M. E. Lidell, M. E. V. Johansson, M. Mörgelin, N. Asker, J. R. Gum, Y. S. Kim, and G. C. Hansson, The recombinant C-terminus of the human MUC2 mucin forms dimers in CHO cells and heterodimers with full-length MUC2 in LS 174T cells, *Biochem. J.* **372**, 335-345 (2002).

8. N. Asker, M. A. B. Axelsson, S. O. Olofsson, and G. C. Hansson, Human MUC5AC mucin dimerizes in the rough endoplasmic reticulum, similarly to the MUC2 mucin, *Biochem. J.* **335**, 381-387 (1998).

9. I. Carlstedt, A. Herrmann, H. Karlsson, J. K. Sheehan, L. Fransson, and G. C. Hansson, Characterization of two different glycosylated domains from the insoluble mucin complex of rat small intestine, *J. Biol. Chem.* **268**, 18771-18781 (1993).

10. A. Herrmann, J. R. Davies, G. Lindell, S. Martensson, N. H. Packer, D. M. Swallow, and I. Carlstedt, Studies on the "Insoluble" glycoprotein complex from human colon, Jou *J. Biol. Chem.* **274**, 15828-15836 (1999).

11. G. Xu, L. J. Huan, I. A. Khatre, D. Wang, A. Bennic, R. E. F. Fahim, G. Forstner, and J. F. Forstner, cDNA for the carboxyl-terminal region of a rat intestinal mucin-like peptide, *J. Biol. Chem.* **267**, 5401-5407 (1992).

12. M. E. Lidell, M. E. V. Johansson, and G. C. Hansson, An autocatalytic cleavage in the C-terminus of the human MUC2 mucin occurs at the low pH of the late secretory pathway, *J. Biol. Chem.* **278**, 13944-13951 (2003).

13. R. R. Parmley and S. J. Gendler, Cystic fibrosis mice lacking Muc1 have reduced amounts of intestinal mucus, *J. Clinical Invest.* **102**, 1798-1806 (1998).

14. M. Hinojosa-Kurtzberg, M. E. V. Johansson, C. S. Madsen, G. C. Hansson, and S. J. Gendler, Novel MUC1 splice variants contribute to mucin over-expression in CFTR deficient mice, *AJP - Gastrointestinal and Liver Physiol.* **284**, G853-G862 (2003).

15. J. D. Li, W. J. Feng, M. Gallup, J. H. Kim, J. Gum, Y. Kim, and C. B. Basbaum, Activation of NF-Kappa-B via a SRC-dependent ras-MAPK-PP90RSK pathway is required for pseudomonas aeruginosa-induced mucin overproduction in epithelial cells, *Proc. Natl. Acad. Sci. U.S.A.* **95**, 5718-5723 (1998).

16. J. R. Davies, N. Svitacheva, L. Lannefors, R. Kornfalt, and I. Carlstedt, Identification of MUC5B, MUC5AC and small amounts of MUC2 mucins in cystic fibrosis airway secretions, *Biochem. J.* **344**, 321-330 (1999).

17. J. D. Li, A. F. Dohrman, M. Gallup, S. Miyata, J. R. Gum, Y. S. Kim, J. A. Nadel, A. Prince, and C. B. Basbaum, Transcriptional activation of mucin by Pseudomonas aeruginosa lipopolysaccharide in the pathogenesis of cystic fibrosis lung disease, *Proc. Natl. Acad. Sci. U.S.A.* **94**, 967-972 (1997).

18. C. Wickstrom, C. Christersson, J. R. Davies, and I. Carlstedt, Macromolecular organization of saliva: Identification of insouble MUC5B assemblies and non-mucin proteins in the gel phase, *Biochem. J.* **351**, 421-428 (2000).

19. R. D. Coakley, B. R. Grubb, A. M. Paradiso, J. T. Gatzy, L. G. Johnson, S. M. Kreda, W. K. Neal, and R. C. Boucher, Abnormal surface liquid pH regulation by cultured cystic fibrosis bronchial epithelium, *Proc. Natl. Acad. Sci. U.S.A.* **100**, 16083-16088 (2003).

Index